Date: 8/23/21

613.2622 RIC
Richer, Alice C.,
Vegetarian and vegan diets :
your questions answered /

D1595624

Vegetarian and Vegan Diets

Recent Titles in
Q&A Health Guides

VEGETARIAN AND VEGAN DIETS

Your Questions Answered

Alice C. Richer

Q&A Health Guides

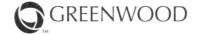

An Imprint of ABC-CLIO, LLC

Santa Barbara, California • Denver, Colorado

Library of Congress Cataloging-in-Publication Data

Names: Richer, Alice C., author.
Title: Vegetarian and vegan diets : your questions answered / Alice C. Richer.
Description: Santa Barbara, California : Greenwood, an imprint of ABC-CLIO, LLC, 2021. | Series: Q&a health guides | Includes bibliographical references and index.
Identifiers: LCCN 2020035089 (print) | LCCN 2020035090 (ebook) | ISBN 9781440870989 (print : acid-free paper) | ISBN 9781440870996 (ebook)
Subjects: LCSH: Vegetarian cooking. | Nutrition
Classification: LCC TX837 .R498 2021 (print) | LCC TX837 (ebook) | DDC 641.5/636—dc23
LC record available at https://lccn.loc.gov/2020035089
LC ebook record available at https://lccn.loc.gov/2020035090

ISBN: 978-1-4408-7098-9 (print)
     978-1-4408-7099-6 (ebook)

25 24 23 22 21   1 2 3 4 5

This book is also available as an eBook.

Greenwood
An Imprint of ABC-CLIO, LLC

ABC-CLIO, LLC
147 Castilian Drive
Santa Barbara, California 93117
www.abc-clio.com

This book is printed on acid-free paper ∞

Manufactured in the United States of America

This book is dedicated to my family.

Contents

Series Foreword

All of us have questions about our health. Is this normal? Should I be doing something differently? Whom should I talk to about my concerns? And our modern world is full of answers. Thanks to the Internet, there's a wealth of information at our fingertips, from forums where people can share their personal experiences to Wikipedia articles to the full text of medical studies. But finding the right information can be an intimidating and difficult task—some sources are written at too high a level, others have been oversimplified, while still others are heavily biased or simply inaccurate.

Q&A Health Guides address the needs of readers who want accurate, concise answers to their health questions, authored by reputable and objective experts, and written in clear and easy-to-understand language. This series focuses on the topics that matter most to young adult readers, including various aspects of physical and emotional well-being as well as other components of a healthy lifestyle. These guides will also serve as a valuable tool for parents, school counselors, and others who may need to answer teens' health questions.

All books in the series follow the same format to make finding information quick and easy. Each volume begins with an essay on health literacy and why it is so important when it comes to gathering and evaluating health information. Next, the top five myths and misconceptions that surround the topic are dispelled. The heart of each guide is a collection of questions and answers, organized thematically. A selection of five case studies provides real-world examples to illuminate key concepts. Rounding out each volume are a directory of resources, glossary, and index.

It is our hope that the books in this series will not only provide valuable information but will also help guide readers toward a lifetime of healthy decision making.

Introduction

Vegetarian and Vegan Diets: Your Questions Answered is dedicated to educating the average person about the many benefits of plant-based diets. Plant-based diets have never been more popular than in recent years, although they have been adhered to since the time of the Egyptians. While it still does not appear that a majority of people follow a diet that eliminates some or all animal foods, the number of people reducing or avoiding meat is estimated to have increased by 70 percent worldwide over the past decade. Individuals are also increasingly demanding meat replacement plant-based foods, which are found more easily in supermarkets and restaurants than ever before. From 2014 to 2017, demand for vegan food products increased by 92 percent in Australia and most westernized countries have seen an increase in demand for meatless food products from 3 percent to 14 percent during 2017–2018.

There are many different variations of plant-based diets, from vegetarian that typically excludes meat but includes dairy foods and eggs, flexitarian and Mediterranean that stress vegetables but allow all animal foods in moderation, to vegan that eliminates all foods and products that are derived from animals. There are many studies discussed in the book that show plant-based diets can help to prevent chronic illnesses or significantly improve the health of those of those who have already developed them. The China study, one of the most well known of these studies, is reviewed in this book and discusses the many health benefits of plant-based diets.

But the nutrition history of the Pima Indian tribe highlights the powerful effects a plant-based diet can have on health. The Pima Indians have a history of excessively high rates of obesity and diabetes of all Americans and have been studied for a number of years. When Pima tribe members who were obese and had diabetes reverted to a plant-based diet tradition-ally eaten by their ancestors, they experienced drastic reductions in their weight, reversal of diabetes, and improvements in health outcomes.

However, not everyone thrives on a plant-based diet, and these diets may also have negative health consequences that many people are unaware of. The most important, and all too common, negative impact comes from improper nutritional planning. When animal foods are removed from the human diet, important nutrients they contain (that are also required for good health) may be unintentionally eliminated. This in turn can result in poor health, weight loss, and nutrient deficiencies. Plant-based meat-less food products are not always healthy food options either, as many people believe. For instance, one current popular meatless food product is the Impossible Burger. It is commonly assumed this product is healthier than a typical beef burger. But nutritionally it is not. As reviewed in this book, the Impossible Burger has 240 calories, 8 grams of saturated fat, and 370 milligrams of sodium in a 4 ounce serving size. In comparison, a 4 oz lean beef hamburger has 170 calories, 3.5 grams of saturated fat, and 75 milligrams of sodium.

Plant-based diets may also have other negative ramifications that many people are unaware of. Some of these include unknown food allergies, intolerances, or sensitivities to foods that were previously eaten sparingly or are new to the diet. Adverse reactions to naturally occurring com-pounds found in plant foods can also have negative effects when some-one overindulges. For example, eating too many phytates (found in many plant foods such as walnuts) can inflame the gastrointestinal tract and contribute to malnutrition because of their ability to decrease nutrient absorption. In addition, while plant foods are a good source of fiber, some individuals have difficulty tolerating it. This poor fiber tolerance can create a number of medical problems and poor health. Plant-based diet choices may also mask an undiagnosed eating disorder. Studies find that individuals predisposed to eating disorders are more likely to follow a veg-etarian meal plan as a socially acceptable way of hiding their disease. This is why accurate nutrition knowledge and planning is so important when following a meatless or reduced meat diet to reap the many health benefits plant-based diets appear to offer. This book is a resource of accurate nutri-tion information written by a registered dietitian to help you, the reader, learn to successfully maintain good health.

Individuals choose to eliminate some, or all, animal foods from their diet for a number of different reasons. The most popular reason is to improve health or prevent chronic diseases. But some individuals choose to follow a plant-based diet to help slow climate change or to support the reduction of cruelty to animals raised for human consumption. No matter what the reason an individual chooses for changing to a plant-based diet, most people who follow them are passionate about their beliefs and their new diet. This passion can sometimes lead to problems with family and friends. This book analyzes some of the reasons people chose to eliminate meat from their diet and provides individuals tools and strategies that are helpful to make the transition to a plant-based way of life easier and acceptable for long-term success and health.

Guide to Health Literacy

On her 13th birthday, Samantha was diagnosed with type 2 diabetes. She consulted her mom and her aunt, both of whom also have type 2 diabetes, and decided to go with their strategy of managing diabetes by taking insulin. As a result of participating in an after-school program at her middle school that focused on health literacy, she learned that she can help manage the level of glucose in her bloodstream by counting her carbohydrate intake, following a diabetic diet, and exercising regularly. But, what exactly should she do? How does she keep track of her carbohydrate intake? What is a diabetic diet? How long should she exercise and what type of exercise should she do? Samantha is a visual learner, so she turned to her favorite source of media, YouTube, to answer these questions. She found videos from individuals around the world sharing their experiences and tips, doctors (or at least people who have "Dr." in their YouTube channel names), government agencies such as the National Institutes of Health, and even video clips from cat lovers who have cats with diabetes. With guidance from the librarian and the health and science teachers at her school, she assessed the credibility of the information in these videos and even compared their suggestions to some of the print resources that she was able to find at her school library. Now, she knows exactly how to count her carbohydrate level, how to prepare and follow a diabetic diet, and how much (and what) exercise is needed daily. She intends to share her findings with her mom and her aunt, and now she wants to create a chart that summarizes what she has learned that she can share with her doctor.

Samantha's experience is not unique. She represents a shift in our society; an individual no longer views himself or herself as a passive recipient of medical care but as an active mediator of his or her own health. However, in this era when any individual can post his or her opinions and experiences with a particular health condition online with just a few clicks or publish a memoir, it is vital that people know how to assess the credibility of health information. Gone are the days when "publishing" health information required intense vetting. The health information landscape is highly saturated, and people have innumerable sources where they can find information about practically any health topic. The sources (whether print, online, or a person) that an individual consults for health information are crucial because the accuracy and trustworthiness of the information can potentially affect his or her overall health. The ability to find, select, assess, and use health information constitutes a type of literacy—health literacy—that everyone must possess.

THE DEFINITION AND PHASES OF HEALTH LITERACY

One of the most popular definitions for health literacy comes from Ratzan and Parker (2000), who describe health literacy as "the degree to which individuals have the capacity to obtain, process, and understand basic health information and services needed to make appropriate health decisions." Recent research has extrapolated health literacy into health literacy bits, further shedding light on the multiple phases and literacy practices that are embedded within the multifaceted concept of health literacy. Although this research has focused primarily on online health information seeking, these health literacy bits are needed to successfully navigate both print and online sources. There are six phases of health information seeking: (1) Information Need Identification and Question Formulation, (2) Information Search, (3) Information Comprehension, (4) Information Assessment, (5) Information Management, and (6) Information Use.

The first phase is the *information need identification and question formulation phase*. In this phase, one needs to be able to develop and refine a range of questions to frame one's search and understand relevant health terms. In the second phase, *information search*, one has to possess appropriate searching skills, such as using proper keywords and correct spelling in search terms, especially when using search engines and databases. It is also crucial to understand how search engines work (i.e., how search results are derived, what the order of the search results means, how to use the snippets that are provided in the search results list to select websites, and how to determine which listings are ads on a search engine results page). One also has to limit reliance on surface characteristics, such as the design of a website or a book (a website or book that appears to have a lot of information or looks aesthetically pleasant does not necessarily mean it has good information) and language used (a website or book that utilizes jargon, the keywords that one used to conduct the search, or the word "information" does not necessarily indicate it will have good information). The next phase is *information comprehension*, whereby one needs to have the ability to read, comprehend, and recall the information (including textual, numerical, and visual content) one has located from the books and/or online resources.

To assess the credibility of health information (*information assessment* phase), one needs to be able to evaluate information for accuracy, evaluate how current the information is (e.g., when a website was last updated or when a book was published), and evaluate the creators of the source—for example, examine site sponsors or type of sites (.com, .gov, .edu, or .org) or the author of a book (practicing doctor, a celebrity doctor, a patient of a specific disease, etc.) to determine the believability of the person/ organization providing the information. Such credibility perceptions tend to become generalized, so they must be frequently reexamined (e.g., the belief that a specific news agency always has credible health information needs continuous vetting). One also needs to evaluate the credibility of the medium (e.g., television, Internet, radio, social media, and book) and evaluate—not just accept without questioning—others' claims regarding the validity of a site, book, or other specific source of information. At this stage, one has to "make sense of information gathered from diverse sources by identifying misconceptions, main and supporting ideas, conflicting information, point of view, and biases" (American Association of School Librarians [AASL], 2009, p. 13) and conclude which sources/ information are valid and accurate by using conscious strategies rather than simply using intuitive judgments or "rules of thumb." This phase is the most challenging segment of health information seeking and serves as a determinant of success (or lack thereof) in the information-seeking process. The following section on Sources of Health Information further explains this phase.

The fifth phase is *information management*, whereby one has to organize information that has been gathered in some manner to ensure easy retrieval and use in the future. The last phase is *information use*, in which one will synthesize information found across various resources, draw conclusions, and locate the answer to his or her original question and/ or the content that fulfills the information need. This phase also often involves implementation, such as using the information to solve a health problem; make health-related decisions; identify and engage in behaviors that will help a person to avoid health risks; share the health information found with family members and friends who may benefit from it; and advocate more broadly for personal, family, or community health.

THE IMPORTANCE OF HEALTH LITERACY

The conception of health has moved from a passive view (someone is either well or ill) to one that is more active and process based (someone is working toward preventing or managing disease). Hence, the dominant focus has shifted from doctors and treatments to patients and prevention, resulting in the need to strengthen our ability and confidence (as patients and consumers of health care) to look for, assess, understand, manage, share, adapt, and use health-related information. An individual's health literacy level has been found to predict his or her health status better than age, race, educational attainment, employment status, and income level (National Network of Libraries of Medicine, 2013). Greater health literacy also enables individuals to better communicate with health care providers such as doctors, nutritionists, and therapists, as they can pose more relevant, informed, and useful questions to health care providers. Another added advantage of greater health literacy is better information-seeking skills, not only for health but also in other domains, such as completing assignments for school.

SOURCES OF HEALTH INFORMATION: THE GOOD, THE BAD, AND THE IN-BETWEEN

For generations, doctors, nurses, nutritionists, health coaches, and other health professionals have been the trusted sources of health information. Additionally, researchers have found that young adults, when they have health-related questions, typically turn to a family member who has had firsthand experience with a health condition because of their family member's close proximity and because of their past experience with, and trust in, this individual. Expertise should be a core consideration when consulting a person, website, or book for health information. The credentials and background of the person or author and conflicting interests of the author (and his or her organization) must be checked and validated to ensure the likely credibility of the health information they are conveying. While books often have implied credibility because of the peer-review process involved, self-publishing has challenged this credibility, so qualifications of book authors should also be verified. When it comes to health information, currency of the source must also be examined. When examining health information/studies presented, pay attention to the exhaustiveness of research methods utilized to offer recommendations or conclusions. Small and nondiverse sample size is often—but not always—an indication of reduced credibility. Studies that confuse correlation with causation is another potential issue to watch for. Information seekers must also pay attention to the sponsors of the research studies. For example, if a study is sponsored by manufacturers of drug Y and the study recommends that drug Y is the best treatment to manage or cure a disease, this may indicate a lack of objectivity on the part of the researchers.

The Internet is rapidly becoming one of the main sources of health information. Online forums, news agencies, personal blogs, social media sites, pharmacy sites, and celebrity "doctors" are all offering medical and health information targeted to various types of people in regard to all types of diseases and symptoms. There are professional journalists, citizen journalists, hoaxers, and people paid to write fake health news on various sites that may appear to have a legitimate domain name and may even have authors who claim to have professional credentials, such as an MD. All these sites *may* offer useful information or information that appears to be useful and relevant; however, much of the information may be debatable and may fall into gray areas that require readers to discern credibility, reliability, and biases.

While broad recognition and acceptance of certain media, institutions, and people often serve as the most popular determining factors to assess credibility of health information among young people, keep in mind that there are legitimate Internet sites, databases, and books that publish health information and serve as sources of health information for doctors, other health sites, and members of the public. For example, MedlinePlus (https://medlineplus.gov) has trusted sources on over 975 diseases and conditions and presents the information in easy-to-understand language.

The chart here presents factors to consider when assessing credibility of health information. However, keep in mind that these factors function only as a guide and require continuous updating to keep abreast with the changes in the landscape of health information, information sources, and technologies.

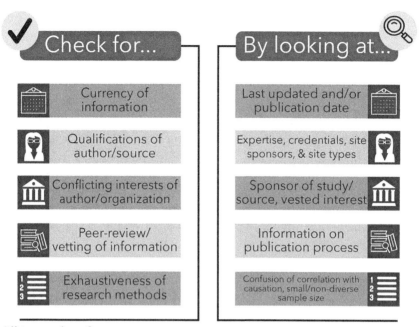

All images from flaticon.com

The chart can serve as a guide; however, approaching a librarian about how one can go about assessing the credibility of both print and online health information is far more effective than using generic checklist-type tools. While librarians are not health experts, they can apply and teach patrons strategies to determine the credibility of health information.

With the prevalence of fake sites and fake resources that appear to be legitimate, it is important to use the following health information assessment tips to verify health information that one has obtained (St. Jean et al., 2015, p. 151):

- **Don't assume you are right**: Even when you feel very sure about an answer, keep in mind that the answer may not be correct, and it is important to conduct (further) searches to validate the information.
- **Don't assume you are wrong**: You may actually have correct information, even if the information you encounter does not match—that is, you may be right and the resources that you have found may contain false information.
- **Take an open approach**: Maintain a critical stance by not including your preexisting beliefs as keywords (or letting them influence your

choice of keywords) in a search, as this may influence what it is possible to find out.

- **Verify, verify, and verify**: Information found, especially on the Internet, needs to be validated, no matter how the information appears on the site (i.e., regardless of the appearance of the site or the quantity of information that is included).

Health literacy comes with experience navigating health information. Professional sources of health information, such as doctors, health care providers, and health databases, are still the best, but one also has the power to search for health information and then verify it by consulting with these trusted sources and by using the health information assessment tips and guide shared previously.

Mega Subramaniam, PhD
Associate Professor, College of Information Studies,
University of Maryland

REFERENCES AND FURTHER READING

American Association of School Librarians (AASL). (2009). *Standards for the 21st-century learner in action*. Chicago, IL: American Association of School Librarians.

Hilligoss, B., & Rieh, S.-Y. (2008). Developing a unifying framework of credibility assessment: Construct, heuristics, and interaction in context. *Information Processing & Management*, 44(4), 1467–1484.

Kuhlthau, C. C. (1988). Developing a model of the library search process: Cognitive and affective aspects. *Reference Quarterly*, 28(2), 232–242.

National Network of Libraries of Medicine (NNLM). (2013). Health literacy. Bethesda, MD: National Network of Libraries of Medicine. Retrieved from nnlm.gov/outreach/consumer/hlthlit.html

Ratzan, S. C., & Parker, R. M. (2000). Introduction. In C. R. Selden, M. Zorn, S. C. Ratzan, & R. M. Parker (Eds.), *National Library of Medicine current bibliographies in medicine: Health literacy*. NLM Pub. No. CBM 2000–1. Bethesda, MD: National Institutes of Health, U.S. Department of Health and Human Services.

St. Jean, B., Taylor, N. G., Kodama, C., & Subramaniam, M. (February 2017). Assessing the health information source perceptions of tweens using card-sorting exercises. *Journal of Information Science*. Retrieved from http://journals.sagepub.com/doi/abs/10.1177/0165551516687728

St. Jean, B., Subramaniam, M., Taylor, N. G., Follman, R., Kodama, C., & Casciotti, D. (2015). The influence of positive hypothesis testing on youths' online health-related information seeking. *New Library World*, *116*(3/4), 136–154.

Subramaniam, M., St. Jean, B., Taylor, N. G., Kodama, C., Follman, R., & Casciotti, D. (2015). Bit by bit: Using design-based research to improve the health literacy of adolescents. *JMIR Research Protocols*, *4*(2), paper e62. Retrieved from http://www.ncbi.nlm.nih.gov/pmc/articles/PMC4464334/

Valenza, J. (2016, November 26). Truth, truthiness, and triangulation: A news literacy toolkit for a "post-truth" world [Web log]. Retrieved from http://blogs.slj.com/neverendingsearch/2016/11/26/truth-truthiness-triangulation-and-the-librarian-way-a-news-literacy-toolkit-for-a-post-truth-world/

Common Misconceptions about Vegetarian and Vegan Diets

1. VEGETARIAN AND VEGAN DIETS ARE BORING AND LACK VARIETY

Most people assume, because plant-based foods tend to be mild in taste, that vegetarian and vegan diets are boring and lack variety and flavor. But that is far from the truth. Many vegetarian and vegan diets can be very flavorful when plant foods are combined with herbs and spices in creative recipes. Many websites and recipe books now cater to vegetarians and vegans with a plethora of interesting, easy to make, and flavorful recipes ready for use. Most supermarkets also carry a wide variety of vegetarian and vegan meals and ingredients, making it much easier to follow a plant-based diet than ever before.

2. PLANT-BASED DIETS ARE EXPENSIVE AND DIFFICULT TO FOLLOW

It is generally assumed that vegetables, legumes, and whole grains are more expensive than animal foods eaten in traditional diets. However, traditional westernized diet plans that include processed foods and animal foods can actually be more expensive over the course of a lifetime. Eating vegetarian and vegan diets may actually reduce food costs because plant-based foods tend to require less food to be satisfying and meet nutritional needs. Switching from a traditional diet to a plant-based diet takes some planning and effort, but once the switch is made, it can be just as economical and easy to follow when compared to a traditional meat-based diet.

3. VEGETARIAN AND VEGAN DIETS WILL RESULT IN NUTRITIONAL DEFICIENCIES

It is true that nutrition deficiencies can occur if a plant-based diet is not planned properly. Vegans and vegetarians who just stop eating all animal foods without proper nutritional planning are often found to develop deficiencies of vitamins B_{12} and D, calcium, heme-iron, omega-3s, riboflavin, zinc, and some amino acids because these nutrients are found almost exclusively in animal-based foods. However, vegans and vegetarians who work with a registered dietitian or those who carefully plan how to eat nutritionally on a plant-based diet can reduce their risk for these common plant-based diet nutrient deficiencies.

4. VEGANS AND VEGETARIANS HAVE A LOWER INCIDENCE OF CHRONIC DISEASES AND ARE HEALTHIER THAN THOSE WHO EAT MEAT

A good number of research studies do indeed find that a plant-based diet lowers the overall risk for cardiovascular disease, diabetes, and other chronic illnesses. Vegetarian and vegan diets may also help individuals to lose weight. However, this is not true for everyone. Individual genetic traits or health of the gastrointestinal microbiome may predispose a person to poor health outcomes when following a plant-based diet. Inadequate diet planning may also increase the risk for poor health and chronic illnesses. It is always important that an individual be assessed by a skilled nutrition professional before starting a vegetarian or vegan diet to ensure proper diet planning to improve or maintain good health.

5. VEGETARIAN AND VEGAN DIETS ARE ALWAYS A HEALTHY OPTION

Removing highly processed animal foods that have high amounts of saturated fats and sodium from the daily diet is always a good nutrition choice that has shown positive impacts on overall health. But while many people assume vegetarian and vegan food choices are much healthier than animal foods, that is not always the case. Many processed plant-based food choices can be just as high in sugar, salt, and saturated fats as animal foods. This is why reading food labels, working with a nutrition professional, or adequately studying and planning a vegetarian or vegan diet prior to following one is so important for improving or maintaining good health.

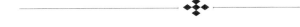

QUESTIONS AND ANSWERS

❖

The Basics

1. What is a plant-based diet?

Most people assume a plant-based diet eliminates all foods from animal sources, such as dairy, eggs, fish, poultry, and red meats. However, while plant foods are the foundation of plant-based diets, animal foods are not always excluded. There are many different variations of plant-based diets. The type of plant-based diet an individual selects is based on their personal motivations. These motivations may be to improve health or to follow moral, environmental, or religious convictions, or a combination of all of these. The most common plant-based meal plans people choose are vegetarian or semivegetarian subtypes (flexitarian, lacto-ovo vegetarian, lactarian, Mediterranean, pescatarian) and vegan.

While the vegetarian diet was the first plant-based diet to become popular during modern times, it is believed that vegetarianism was first put into practice as far back as 3200 BCE. The practice of vegetarianism was popular among many religious groups in ancient Egypt. Pythagoreans, individuals who supported the theories of the Greek philosopher Pythagoras, were among the first self-proclaimed vegetarians. Pythagoras, known as the first mathematician who influenced Western philosophy, moved to Egypt in 580 BCE. He taught his pupils that animals should be treated kindly and that abstinence from meat was important for the human soul. Other ancient Greek philosophers, including Plato and Socrates, also endorsed vegetarian diets. Ancient religious sects of the time (Buddhists, Brahmans,

Hindus, and Zoroastrians) expected their followers to eat a vegetarian diet to conform to the religious belief that all living creatures should be treated with compassion. Vegetarian diets continued to be popular in medieval Europe from the fifth century to the fifteenth century. Some well-known vegetarians were St. Francis of Assisi (1181–1226), Leonardo Da Vinci (1452–1519), and John Locke (1632–1704). Compassion and kindness for animals and health benefits were the motivating factors cited by these individuals for following a vegetarian diet. By the 1800s, vegetarian restaurants were popular in London, and the Vegetarian Society was founded in 1847. The International Vegetarian Union (IVU) was born in 1908 in Dresden, Germany, to support global vegetarianism. During World War II (1939–45), vegetarian diets became the norm due to acute food shortages, especially for meat. A nationwide effort encouraging British citizens to grow their own fruits and vegetables and follow a vegetarian meal plan sustained the British population throughout the war years.

Plant-based diets were also common in the United States. Sylvester Graham (1794–1851), a Bostonian clergyman, promoted vegetarian diets for health and religious reasons. But it wasn't until the 1970s that vegetarian diets really began to gain popularity in the United States. In 1971, Frances Moore Lappé published *Diet for a Small Planet*. She promoted plant-based, meatless diets, although eggs and dairy foods were allowed. Lappé's motivation for promoting a plant-based diet was both environmental, due to the negative environmental impact of meat production techniques, and political, due to the belief that population growth would worsen food shortages and malnutrition over time.

Transitioning from animal-based diets to plant-based diets can be difficult for some people. As a result, numerous variations of vegetarian meal plans were developed and are known as semivegetarian diets. The most popular semivegetarian diets are lacto-ovo, lactarian, and pescatarian. All of these alternate versions of a vegetarian diet include the foundation of plant foods and elimination of red meats (beef, lamb, pork) and poultry.

The term "flexitarian" emerged in 2014 as a flexible vegetarian diet for those who want to eat healthier but do not necessarily want to be a vegetarian or vegan. Flexitarians are also considered to be semivegetarians. The flexitarian meal plan considers meat to be an important source of protein, fat, and micronutrients, but it recognizes that an excess amount of meat consumption is detrimental for health. Some flexitarians also choose this diet because of personal concerns about the ethical treatment of animals and the environment.

An alternate, and stricter, version of a vegetarian or semivegetarian meal plan is the vegan diet. Vegans do not eat any foods that come from animal sources, and all of their food choices are plant-based. But veganism is also a way of life because it excludes the use of any clothing or personal care products from animals and insects, such as bees. Vegan meal plans can be traced back to as early as 500 BCE and are included in the history of vegetarianism. This way of life began to formalize into the vegan diet by 1806, based on the beliefs of Dr. William Lambe (1765–1848). Dr. Lambe, for personal health reasons, changed his diet to include only beans, fruits, grains, nuts, seeds, vegetables, and distilled water. In his 1815 book *Water and Vegetable Diet in Consumption, Scrofula, Cancer, Asthma, and Other Chronic Diseases*, Dr. Lambe stated, "My reason for objecting to every species of matter to be used as food, except the direct produce of the earth—as may be seen in my last publication—is founded on the broad ground that no other matter is suited to the organs of man. This applies then with the same force to eggs, milk, cheese, and fish, as to flesh meat." John Frank Newton, a patient of Dr. Lambe's, expanded upon the health reasons for the diet to include the ethical treatment of animals.

The Vegan Society credits Donald Watson as the founder of the vegan diet movement in 1944. Watson, along with six other vegetarians, founded the Vegan Society, and all were "nondairy" vegetarians. They coined the term "vegan" using the first three and last two letters of the word "vegetarian." In 1949, Leslie J. Cross defined the term "veganism" as "to seek an end to the use of animals by man for food, commodities, work, hunting, vivisection, and by all other uses involving exploitation of animal life by man."

Many vegans choose this diet plan because of their moral and ethical convictions regarding the reported maltreatment of animals raised for human consumption. *Introduction to Animal Rights* by Gary L. Francione and *Eat Like You Care* by Anna Charlton, both staunch vegans, are two tomes that detail how animals are used for food, clothing, and entertainment. Vegans feel strongly that animals should not be harmed. The International Vegan Association (IVA) defines a vegan as "someone with a lived commitment to not use or consume animals or animal products for any purpose, including food (e.g., dairy, honey, meat, bone-char refined sugar, eggs), clothing (e.g., silk, leather, wool), and entertainment (e.g., animal racing, hunting)."

The concept of sustainability of the food supply for human consumption is another important concern to many people worldwide that has also increased the interest in plant-based diets. The Food and Agriculture Organization (FAO) of the United Nations define sustainable diets as "those diets with low environmental impacts that contribute to food and nutrition security and to healthy life for present and future generations.

Sustainable diets are protective and respectful of biodiversity and ecosystems, culturally acceptable, accessible, economically fair and affordable, nutritionally adequate, safe, and healthy, while optimizing natural and human resources."

2. What are the different types of plant-based diets?

While there is no standard definition of what a plant-based diet is, it is typically defined as a daily meal plan whose foundation is built on foods from plant sources. Common plant food sources are avocados, beans, fresh fruits, fresh herbs, legumes, nuts and seeds, olives and olive oil, poly- and monounsaturated oils, nuts and seeds, spices, vegetables, and whole grains. Foods from animals, such as dairy, eggs, fish, poultry, and red meats, are either allowed in limited amounts or eliminated, depending upon the beliefs or goals of the individual following the diet. All plant-based diet variations limit the amount of sweets and sugar allowed. The most popular variations of plant-based diets include flexitarian, Mediterranean, pescatarian, vegetarian or semivegetarian, vegan, and whole-food, plant-based, low-fat meal plans. Other less popular versions are raw food vegan diets.

The type of plant-based diet an individual chooses to follow depends upon the beliefs and goals of that individual. Most people switch to a plant-based diet for health reasons. Numerous studies show health benefits and improved health outcomes, such as lower blood pressure, reduced diabetes and heart disease progression, and cancer prevention when plant-based diets are followed. Individuals may also change to a plant-based diet because they are concerned about the environment or wish to comply with religious doctrines.

As discussed in Question 1, plant-based diets do not always eliminate animal foods. Vegetarian diets typically eliminate eggs, dairy, fish, meat, and poultry, but there are numerous variations of the vegetarian meal plan. Known as semivegetarian diets, lacto-ovo vegetarian diets allow eggs and dairy foods. Lactarian meal plans eliminate eggs but allow dairy foods. The pescatarian meal plan allows fish but no other animal foods.

Another semivegetarian meal plan, and one of the most popular, is the Mediterranean diet. It is often recommended for improved health because of verified health benefits from numerous studies and because it is a diet that most people can realistically follow for the rest of their lives. The Mediterranean meal plan represents the cultural and traditional dietary patterns of individuals who live in countries that border the Mediterranean Sea. The diet itself emphasizes consuming foods primarily from plants but does include dairy, eggs, fish, poultry, and occasional red meat in moderation. The core foods of the Mediterranean diet are rich in anti-oxidants and unsaturated fats and this diet is usually selected for health reasons. This diet is explored in depth in Question 3.

Created by dietitian Dawn Jackson Blatner, the flexitarian diet is more flexible in what foods are allowed, as the name implies. Another semiveg-etarian diet plan, the flexitarian meal plan claims to provide the health benefits of a vegetarian diet while including limited amounts of animal foods. The foundation of this diet includes fruits, legumes, vegetables, protein from plant foods, and whole grains. But it also occasionally allows dairy, eggs, fish, meat, and seafood. Sugars, sweets, and processed foods are discouraged. The flexitarian meal plan is appealing because it makes it easier for an individual to transition from a traditional meat-based diet to a more plant-based meal plan, while also emphasizing healthier food choices and the flexibility to include some meat.

Pescatarian diets include plant-based foods, but protein foods are sup-plied primarily from fish and seafood, preferably wild caught. A pesca-tarian is defined in the Merriam-Webster dictionary as "one whose diet includes fish but no other meat." However, some pescatarians do include dairy and eggs in their diet. Pescatarian diets are shown in studies to lower the risk of cancer, diabetes, heart disease, and high blood pressure.

Vegan diets are similar to vegetarian diets because they eliminate most foods that originate from an animal. But vegan diets differ from the vege-tarian diet because it is a way of life that extends into how a person lives and the impact their life has on the lives of animals. A vegan meal plan only allows plant-based foods. All animal products are eliminated from the diet as well as clothing, personal care products, and entertainment choices.

Raw food vegan diets follow the vegan meal plan but exclude all foods cooked at temperatures greater than 118 degrees Fahrenheit. Cooking tem-perature is kept low due to the belief that this will preserve the nutrition content of the food, which is decreased at higher cooking temperatures.

Whole-food, plant-based, low-fat diets encourage eating foods that are minimally processed and in their natural form. Decreased total amounts of nuts and seeds and animal protein in the daily diet are recommended to minimize total fat intake. This is one plant-based diet that has been increasing in popularity.

3. What is a Mediterranean diet, and how does it differ from a plant-based diet?

Mediterranean meal plans are considered plant-based diets, although they do allow animal foods. The daily diet of those living along the

Mediterranean Sea is where the Mediterranean diet originated. These countries include Albania, Algeria, Bosnia, Croatia, Cyprus, Egypt, France, Greece, Herzegovina, Israel, Italy, Lebanon, Libya, Malta, Monaco, Montenegro, Morocco, Slovenia, Spain, Syria, Tunisia, and Turkey. It is difficult to pinpoint when the Mediterranean diet first came into existence. However, it is surmised that it evolved from the time of the Assyrians, Babylonians, Greeks, Persians, Romans, and Sumerians because the eating habits of these cultures centered on the agrarian and religious practices of their time. Bread, wine, and oil were the primary staple foods of these cultures, but the diet was further supplemented with cheese made from sheep milk, fish, seafood, and vegetables. Red meat was still eaten, but in small amounts and infrequently.

Individuals living along the Mediterranean Sea are considered some of the healthiest populations in the world. The Mediterranean meal plan emphasizes consuming whole grains (bread, couscous, pasta, polenta, rice), fish, fruit, legumes, nuts, olives and olive oil, vegetables, and yogurt. Cheese, dairy, eggs, poultry, and occasional red meat are included, but in moderation. Foods in this meal plan are rich in antioxidants, fiber, and unsaturated fats. Complex carbohydrate foods, such as whole-grain breads and pasta, fruit, brown rice, polenta, and vegetables, provide 55–60 percent of the total daily calories a person eats. Ten to fifteen percent of daily calories are chosen from protein foods, 60 percent of which are from animal origins such as fish, poultry, and seafood. Healthy fats, such as from avocados, nuts, olives, oils, and seeds, make up 25–30 percent of daily calories.

American scientist Ancel Keys is credited with the discovery of the numerous health benefits of the Mediterranean diet. Keys identified a correlation between cardiovascular diet outcomes and the Mediterranean diet by comparing the health status of poor populations in small towns of Italy with the wealthier citizens of New York. He found that poor Italians were significantly healthier than wealthy New Yorkers. Keys focused on their diet as the origin for this health discrepancy. This focus evolved into the Seven Countries Study. The Seven Countries Study investigated the diet and lifestyle of individuals living in Finland, Greece, Holland, Italy, Japan, the United States, and Yugoslavia in relation to cardiovascular disease incidence using cross-sectional studies.

Cross-sectional studies are also known as observational studies. This means researchers observe their subjects and record specific information about their behaviors in relation to what they are studying, without changing anything in their study subjects' environment or daily life. Cross-sectional studies are chosen as a method to compare different population groups during one specific point in time. The benefit of using a cross-sectional study design is that it allows the observation of many different variables at the same time. These studies do not, however, provide clear-cut information about the cause and effect of the behaviors observed.

Results from the Seven Countries Study scientifically verified positive nutritional and health benefits for those cultures that embraced the Mediterranean way of eating. The population of these countries had significantly lower rates of cholesterol and minimal risk for heart disease. Plentiful use of olive oil, whole-grain breads and pasta, vegetables, fruits, herbs, garlic, red onions, and moderate use of meat represented the core diet of residents living in the countries studied. Many subsequent studies have since verified the numerous health benefits the Mediterranean diet confers upon those who follow it, and it is one of the most well-researched diets to date. However, it should be noted that diet is not the only factor associated with improved health in these cultures. Lifestyle choices, such as exercise frequency, overweight status, and tobacco use, also impacted health outcomes. Lifestyle choices appear to have just as much of an impact on health as diet choices do.

The main difference between Mediterranean and most plant-based diets is the fact that the Mediterranean meal plan allows animal sources of protein from eggs, dairy foods, fish, and some meat. While there is no universal definition of what a plant-based diet is, the foundation of plant-based diets includes fruit, legumes, oils, olives, nuts and seeds, vegetables, and whole grains with an emphasis on plant proteins. But all variations of plant-based diets also support a daily diet that minimizes or eliminates processed foods, added sugars, and genetically modified foods (GMO).

Oldways Preservation Trust, a Boston-based organization that specializes in educating the public about the Mediterranean diet, developed a Mediterranean Diet Pyramid and offers consumers Mediterranean recipes and meal plans.

4. How many people in the United States and worldwide follow a plant-based diet, and are these diets becoming more popular?

It is difficult to accurately assess how many people worldwide actually follow a plant-based diet, but there is statistical data available to help identify them. The United States and Europe survey citizens periodically about their eating habits. There are also many polling companies that research statistics on a variety of societal issues. Some of the more reputable companies that are often cited, and whose data will be examined here, include Gallup, GlobalData, Mintel, the U.S. National Health and Nutrition Examination Survey (NHANES), and Statista. All focus on different areas of research, which makes it difficult to truly determine the actual number of people who engage in a specific activity. However, their data does provide a good indication of societal trends, be it environmental, health, nutrition, or political.

Gallup is an analytics and advice firm that is well known for its surveys on a variety of political and societal issues. Gallup's survey methods are based on telephone interviews with a random sample of adults, aged 18 and older, living in all 50 states in the United States and the District of Columbia. Interview participants are selected using random-digit-dial methods. GlobalData is a consulting and market research company that investigates global trends in many industries for businesses and governments using various research techniques and expert analysis. Mintel describes itself as the "world's leading market intelligence agency" conducting market research, market analysis, and product intelligence of global markets. While methodology varies depending on the country being studied, they primarily use consumer, social media, desk, and trade research techniques along with statistical forecasting methods to forecast product and consumer trends. The U.S. Centers for Disease Control and Prevention (CDC) periodically conducts the NHANES to examine demographics and health behaviors of U.S. citizens. Extensive interviews and medical examinations are conducted every two years for approximately 5,000 civilian and nonincarcerated U.S. citizens. Statista, another market research and consumer data firm that studies consumer trends in the marketplace, analyzes 400 different industries in more than 40 countries using a forecasting model that focuses on revenue trends. Statista uses well-known and reliable classification systems for their analysis, including the North American Industry Classification System (NAICS), the UK Standard Industrial Classification (UK SIC), and the Statistical Classification of Economic Activities in the European Community (NACE Rev 2).

Gallup first began polling Americans about their nutrition habits in 1999. All of their data is based on self-reported information supplied by study participants and is not independently verified. In 1999, Gallup found 6 percent of Americans self-identified as vegetarians. Vegans were not separately distinguished in the first polling data on this subject. However, vegans were included in the 2012 poll, and Gallup found 5 percent of Americans self-identified as vegetarians and 2 percent self-identified as vegans. A 2018 Gallup poll about plant-based diets found that 5 percent of all Americans self-identified as vegetarian and 3 percent as vegan. Gallup further identified that the majority of self-identified vegetarians and vegans ranged between the ages of 18 and 49. Both groups were also more likely to self-identify as being liberal minded and had an annual income of less than $30,000.

While it appears that vegan and vegetarian diets are on the rise worldwide, Gallup results indicate that there has been very little change in the number of individuals in the United States who follow vegetarian or vegan diets between 1999 and 2018. However, although the number of Americans following vegan or vegetarian diets is small compared to the total U.S. population, Gallup found sales of plant-based foods grew by 8 percent during 2017 and exceeded $3.1 billion in sales. This increase in sales of plant-based foods without a concurrent increase in self-reported vegan or vegetarian lifestyle indicates that Americans are increasingly interested in consuming meat alternatives at meals but are not necessarily yet willing to abandon meat from their diet completely.

The NHANES first began collecting self-reported information about health and nutrition in 1999. Questions about vegetarian diets using two 24-hour diet recall interviews were added to the 2007–8 and 2009–10 surveys. The most recent published NHANES survey data about vegetarians, completed in 2007, found that approximately 2 percent of U.S. citizens self-identified as vegetarian and were more likely to be female and college educated and identify as white non-Hispanic or "other" (not black or Hispanic). Fifty-two percent of these self-identified vegetarians reported they still ate meat or fish, and 1 percent did not eat any meat. This seems to indicate that the number of estimated vegetarians in the United States is most likely smaller than expected. The fact that plant-based diets are still not the favored meal plan to follow in the United States is verified by the 2015–2020 NHANES surveys. Results from these surveys found that 75 percent of Americans consume a diet that is suboptimal for dairy, fruit, oil, and vegetable recommendations yet excessive in sugar, saturated fats, and sodium. More than half meet or exceed total grain and total protein recommendations, with the majority of chosen protein sources from animal foods.

In 2018, Statista studied consumers in the United States who self-identified as flexitarians, vegetarians, and vegans, classifying them by generation. They found 5 percent of Americans self-identified as vegetarians and 3 percent as vegans. They further found that the majority of these self-identified vegetarians and vegans were more likely to be between the ages of 18 and 49 and 63 percent of them reported they were flexitarian.

Eight percent of both Gen Y or millennials (born 1980–1994) and Gen Z (born 1995–2015) who self-identified as vegetarians also reported they had totally eliminated meat from their diets.

Outside of the United States, vegan and vegetarian lifestyles appear to be more popular. Statista reported in 2007 that 10–14 percent of young adults in Germany identified as vegetarians or vegans. In the United Kingdom, 3 percent of individuals, aged 19–64 years, followed a vegetarian or vegan diet from 2008 and 2012. In 2015/2016, approximately 11 percent of Western Australians identified as vegetarians. In 2016, 30 percent of Italians included more vegetarian foods in their diet in comparison to 27 percent of French consumers. As of 2016, Asia Pacific had the largest share of vegan consumers globally, with 9 percent of the total population identifying as vegans. As of February 2019, 2 percent of Canadians were identified as vegetarian and 1 percent as vegan. Statista forecasts China, the United Arab Emirates, and Australia to be the fastest-growing markets for vegan food products between 2015 and 2020.

Mintel authored the 2017 Global Food and Drink Trend report, *Power to the Plants*. Their research found that 80 percent of millennials in the United States were more likely to eat meat alternatives some of the time when compared with other age groups. Forty percent of millennials also anticipated purchasing more vegetarian foods in the future when compared to 33 percent of all the other U.S. consumers who expected to do the same. Almost 50 percent of the U.S. consumers cite health concerns as the main reason they consider changing to a plant-based diet. Heart health and weight management were cited as the primary motivators for eating plant-based diets, and 60 percent of the U.S. consumers expressed interest in eating more meat alternatives in their daily diet.

Further research by Mintel, in 2018, found vegan food product offerings in the United Kingdom increased 52 percent between 2014 and 2018 and plant-based protein sales rose by 22 percent between 2013 and 2018. An estimated 26 percent of consumers in the United Kingdom reported they preferred meat-free products; however, Mintel estimates that 90 percent of citizens in the United Kingdom still continue to eat red meat and poultry. However, researchers also found that 34 percent of meat eaters decreased their meat consumption in 2018, especially among British citizens aged 25–34. Thirty-two percent ate less meat to improve health, 31 percent to save money, and 25 percent to support environmental issues.

In Australia, Mintel found vegan product offerings increased 92 percent from 2014 to 2017. Mintel also concluded that Germany is the leader of the "vegan revolution." Vegan food products offered in Germany increased by 240 percent from July 2013 to June 2018. A 2018 Mintel research study concluded that Germany had the highest share of vegan food and drink new product launches between July 2017 and June 2018. Five percent of product offerings were vegan and 11 percent vegetarian. The top countries that show the highest share of global vegan food and drink product launches between July 2017 and June 2018 were Germany (15 percent), United Kingdom (14 percent), United States of America (12 percent), France (4 percent), Spain (4 percent), Australia (3 percent), Italy (3 percent), Canada (3 percent), Austria (3 percent), and Brazil (3 percent). This data indicates that there is an increasing global interest in plant-based meat alternatives, but not necessarily a total shift to a vegan or vegetarian lifestyle. Mintel also surmised that flexitarianism is gaining in popularity, especially in Germany. Twenty percent of Germans, aged 16–24 years old, purchased meat alternatives in 2017. Fifty percent of German consumers report that they believe plant proteins are just as nutritious as animal proteins and 17 percent believe plant proteins taste better than animal proteins.

GlobalData reported in their June 2017 publication, *Top Trends in Prepared Foods 2017: Exploring Trends in Meat, Fish and Seafood; Pasta, Noodles and Rice; Prepared Meals; Savoy Deli Food; Soup; and Meat Substitutes*, that 26 percent of Germans ate a diet reduced in animal proteins in 2014. This increased to 44 percent by 2017. GlobalData also found that 6 percent of Americans claimed to be vegan, an increase of 1 percent from 2014, and 70 percent of people worldwide are reducing or avoiding meat in their daily diet. They concluded millennials are the leaders of this "meatless" movement.

All of these statistics can be very confusing and make it difficult to truly determine how many people eat a plant-based diet. What does appear to be clear, however, is that the majority of people worldwide continue to eat diets that include animal proteins. However, environmental or health-related reasons are influencing an increasing number of people, especially those between the ages of 18 and 49, to seek out plant-based meat alternatives and consider a flexitarian diet option to more closely meet their needs, beliefs, and concerns.

5. What concerns about animals might motivate an individual to change to a plant-based diet?

Concern about the inhumane treatment of animals, animal rights, and animal welfare are some of the primary motivators cited when an individual decides to follow a vegan or vegetarian diet. Faunalytics, a "nonprofit research organization dedicated to helping animals by providing useful information to advocates," conducted a research study of 329 current and former vegans in Germany in 2014 to learn some of the reasons they chose a meatless diet. According to Faunalytics research, 89 percent of survey respondents listed animals as the primary reason for choosing a vegan life-style. Another Faunalytics review found that 50 percent of respondents believed farm animals deserve the same consideration as pets and 16 per-cent bought meat or dairy products labeled "humane."

Vegan and vegetarian societies list animal welfare as the primary rea-son to adopt these lifestyles and diets. The *Vegan Starter Kit*, published by the IVA, states that "it's wrong to harm animals without good reason" and that "we should all be vegan." "Animal rights" are defined by the Vegetarian Resource Group as the belief that nonhuman animals have the basic rights of freedom to "live a natural life from human exploita-tion, unnecessary pain and suffering, and premature death." They define "animal welfare" as the wish to "alleviate the suffering of animals while they are being exploited—without attempting to question the fundamen-tal basis of whether it is acceptable to exploit animals in the first place."

The animal protection movement first began during the early nine-teenth century in the United Kingdom. The prohibition of bull bait-ing, a common sport of dog fighting at that time, was the first legislative bill introduced in the UK Parliament in 1800. In 1822, Colonel Rich-ard Martin succeeded in passing a bill that prevented cruelty to large domestic horses and cattle and founded the Society for the Prevention of Cruelty to Animals (SPCA). Henry Bergh, an American diplomat to Russia, founded the American chapter of the SPCA in New York in 1866. Numerous chapters of the SPCA were subsequently started throughout the United States with the mission to enforce animal anticruelty laws. The SPCAs subsequently expanded to include animal shelters. The American Humane Association (AHA) was founded in 1877 and became the leading national advocate in the United States offering animal and child protection services.

As scientific research and agricultural techniques progressed, concern over the treatment of animals increased with opposition growing toward medical laboratory animal research. The Cruelty to Animals Act, the first antivivisection law, was passed in 1876 in England. Antivivisection is opposition to operating on live animals for scientific research purposes. The AntiVivisection Society was founded in Philadelphia in 1883. Follow-ing World War II, agricultural techniques progressed from agrarian tech-niques to intensive farming methods that increased crop yields and meat production necessary to feed the increasing population of factory workers living in cities. As intensive animal farming methods have evolved, sub-optimal living conditions, feeding practices, and slaughter techniques for animals were exposed. Concern over the treatment of animals raised for food prompted the first federal law in the United States, the Humane Slaughter Act, in 1958. The Humane Slaughter Act, updated in 1978, requires the proper and humane treatment of all animals processed in U.S. Department of Agriculture (USDA) slaughter plants. However, this regulation does not apply to chickens or other birds used for food. There are currently no regulations in the United States that enforce humane treatment of poultry animals, although some individual states have enacted laws protecting them. The Laboratory Animal Welfare Act (1966), the Endangered Species Act (1969), the Horse Protection Act (1970), and the Marine Mammal Protection Act (1972) are all federal laws subsequently passed in the United States for the protection of animals.

Animal protection concerns evolved into the Animal Rights Movement during the 1970s and continues to grow today. Organizations such as People for the Ethical Treatment of Animals (PETA) and Greenpeace emerged as militant animal rights groups that protested against the use of animals for cosmetic and medical research as well as cruel treatment of farm animals. A balanced review of the animal rights movement is presented in the 1998 book *Animal Rights: History and Scope of a Radical Social Movement* by Harold D. Guither. Jim Mason and Peter Singer provide a summary review of factory farming methods and the treatment of animals in their 1980 book *Animal Factories*.

6. What are the environmental factors that might influence an individual to transition to a vegetarian or vegan diet?

Individuals who have environmental concerns frequently choose a vegetarian or vegan lifestyle because of their belief that meat consumption has a bigger impact on the environment and climate change than plant foods do. The 2015 Dietary Guidelines Advisory Committee, established by the U.S. Department of Health and Human Services and the U.S. Department of Agriculture, published a scientific report citing evidence that a plant-based diet with few animal foods was associated with less damage to the environment. The committee found the average diet in the United States, which includes meat and dairy foods, produced more greenhouse gas emissions and used more natural resources than those required for the production of plant-based foods.

Environmentalists, defined as those who are concerned about or advocate for the protection of the environment, are concerned about global warming. Global warming is the theory that the average global temperature has increased at the fastest rate in the past 50 years since global temperatures have been recorded. Global warming is thought to occur when greenhouse gases (water vapor, carbon dioxide, methane, nitrous oxide, and ozone) and air pollutants collect in the atmosphere. As these collect, they absorb sunlight and solar radiation as they bounce off the earth's surface. This in turn prevents these pollutants from escaping into space, which then heats the planet and makes it hotter. It is thought these hotter temperatures are linked to extreme weather events, melting glaciers, rising sea levels, destruction of agriculture and fisheries, disruption of animal habits, and an increase in allergies, asthma, and infectious diseases. Greenhouse gases are produced when fossil fuels are burned, as during transportation (cars, planes, ships, trains, trucks), electricity production, industrial production, agriculture, and land use.

Faunalytics, a nonprofit research organization discussed in Question 5, reported in its February 2019 report, "Climate Change and Animal Agriculture: A Three Step Plan for Policy Makers," that a number of nations pledged to reduce their greenhouse gas (GHG) emissions by the end of the twenty-first century. Climate change advocates argue that food production must be shifted from animal to plant-based foods in order to achieve lower GHG goals. The UN estimates approximately 16 percent of global GHG emissions are attributed to food and agricultural sources, specifically 6 percent from cow meat, 4 percent from cow milk, 1 percent from pig meat, 1 percent from chicken meat, and 4 percent from other sources. Because of this prevailing belief, environmental activists advocate a shift from animal-based to plant-based diets as one method to slow climate change. However, the theory of human-made climate change remains very controversial. Unfortunately, the lack of objective data about it has prompted a passionate disagreement between "climate alarmists" and "climate deniers" with little debate that has led to confusion for the average person.

To understand this whole debate, it is important to understand the agriculture system. Agriculture is the process of plant cultivation and the raising of livestock to produce food for human and animal consumption. In caveman days, humans were hunter-gathers, which meant they collected wild plant-based foods as the staples of their diet and hunted animals for meat. As humans evolved, agriculture shifted toward the cultivation of crops and raising farm animals specifically for food. Individuals often grew their own crops and raised their own animals to meet their own family needs. However, the industrial revolution and technological advances changed an agrarian society from community farming to a society that needed farmers to increase food production and transport it to large population centers, where individuals moved for jobs. Demand for a consistent and safe food supply system grew significantly during the 1800s. Small grocery markets emerged, later evolving into large supermarkets that are common today. Over the past few decades, there has been a return to individuals growing their own crops or raising animals for personal consumption, small farm stands, and farmer markets. However, the majority of global populations continue to purchase the majority of their foods from small and large grocery stores that supply foods from all over the world.

The evolution of agricultural practices has produced a safe food supply with significantly increased crop production to meet increasing population needs. But agricultural practices are very resource intensive, requiring water, electricity, and land with associated transportation costs using fossil fuels. In addition, the use of pesticides to protect crops from insect damage and to increase crop yields is a common practice. To meet the huge global demand for food, large farming operations and animal feedlot and slaughterhouses are needed. It is estimated that agriculture accounts for 28–40 percent of land use worldwide, of which 31 percent is used for crop production and 69 percent for managed pasturelands.

The U.S. Environmental Protection Agency (EPA) reported, in its February 2019 *Draft Inventory of U.S. Greenhouse Gas Emissions*, that agriculture accounted for approximately 8–9 percent of total GHG emissions, with 42 percent of GHG coming from livestock and 50 percent from crop cultivation. One interesting aspect of the GHG debate is the fact that meat production produces a higher percentage of GHG methane than GHG carbon dioxide. Methane is surmised to have a greater impact on global warming than carbon dioxide; however, it also has a half-life that is significantly lower than carbon dioxide. This means it is more quickly removed from the environment. Methane can also be captured and used to produce electricity as a renewable energy source, possibly helping to reduce GHG emissions.

While the agricultural production of meat is often cited as the most detrimental to the environment, cultivation of plant foods can also have their own negative environmental impact. One well-known example of the negative consequences some plant-based crops have is the production of almonds. One individual almond requires 1.1 gallons of water to grow, and 1,900 gallons of water is required to grow one pound of almonds. Approximately 80 percent of almonds are grown in California, and it is estimated that California uses 80 million gallons of water, or 10 percent of its total water supply, annually to grow almond crops. California has experienced drought conditions for a number of years, and it is possible the water needs of almond crops could be worsening drought conditions, having negative impacts for all Californians. It is also estimated that approximately two-thirds of water is used for irrigation of plant crops. Water is a critical environmental resource for the survival of humans and animals. As can be seen, even though agricultural production of meat appears to increase GHGs more than plant crops, plant crops require more water that can reduce the available water needed for survival. In addition, fertilizers and pesticides necessary for better crop yields have their own negative health consequences that must be taken into consideration. Over 3 million tons of pesticides are used annually on crops. As of 1998, 37 million metric tons of chemical fertilizers were used to grow crops. While pesticides and fertilizers can increase crop yields, they are also associated with soil and water contaminations and linked to birth defects, poisoning, and cancers.

A new technique of cultured meats (credited to H. L. Tuomisto and M. J. de Mattos), which are meat products produced in a lab setting using tissue engineering techniques, is reported to produce 74– 96 percent less GHG emissions and use less energy, land, and water compared to conventional European meat production methods. However, while this may be an answer to reducing GHG, cultured meats have yet to be studied for long-term health impacts on humans. One study in 2019 evaluated the impact plant-based meat alternatives could have on the environment. Soy and buckwheat meat alternatives were evaluated for land and water use, GHG emissions, and nitrogen fertilizer run off (a source of pollution). This study estimated nitrogen fertilizer and GHG emissions could be decreased by 35–50 percent, but water use would increase by 15 percent. GHG emissions were reduced by 5 percent.

The climate change debate has led to the reducetarian movement, credited to founder Brian Kateman in 2017. Reducetarians believe that overconsumption of animal agricultural products leads to the destruction of the environment, poor treatment of animals, increases health risks, and contributes to global world hunger. Unlike the beliefs of vegan societies, small changes are encouraged to help animals and the planet. Reducetarians do not believe in an all or nothing approach, but rather a reduction in animal consumption that is comfortable and acceptable to the individual. Eating less red meat, poultry, eggs, and seafood is encouraged, but reducetarians welcome vegans and vegetarians in their movement as well.

7. Do religious or cultural factors influence plant-based diet choices?

Six major religious groups either require or suggest eating a plant-based diet as an important tenet of the faith. These are Buddhism, Christianity, Hinduism, Jainism, Judaism, and Taoism. These faiths vary in core beliefs and whether they follow monotheistic, polytheistic, or nontheistic principles. Monotheistic religions believe in only one God. Polytheistic religions believe in many different gods. Nontheistic religions have no official deity or god. Vegetarianism and religion are the most strongly intertwined in Asian culture. The major faiths of South Asia, and also some of the oldest dating back to ancient India, are Buddhism, Hinduism, and Jainism.

Buddhism, a nontheistic religion, originated from the teachings of Siddhartha Gautama, known as the Buddha or "Awakened One," and spread from India to Central and Southeast Asia, China, Korea, and Japan. Gautama, the son of a warrior king in India, renounced his worldly possessions to become a monk and lived in northern India between the sixth and fourth centuries BCE. He taught four Noble Truths and the Eight-Fold Path as the core principles of Buddhist beliefs. The Noble Truths address the suffering of humanity. The First Noble Truth identifies the presence of suffering in the world. The Second Noble Truth tries to determine the origin of suffering, which is frequently identified as the desire and ignorance of man. The Third Noble Truth stipulates that suffering ends only when one reaches Nirvana. The state of Nirvana is achieved when spiritual enlightenment has been achieved. The Fourth Noble Truth outlines the way to reach Nirvana to end suffering by following the Eight-Fold Path. The Eight-Fold Path is comprised of eight steps: Right Understanding, Right Thought, Right Speech (good moral conduct), Right Action, Right Livelihood, Right Effort (meditation and mental development), Right Mindfulness, and Right Concentration (wisdom or insight). Because the focus of Buddhism is kindness, compassion, and equality, it is stressed that living things should not be killed and life is to be saved and protected. Therefore, practicing Buddhists are strongly encouraged to follow a vegetarian diet. However, unlike some other religions, meat is not expressly prohibited from the diet because of the difficulty some individuals have in giving it up in their diet.

Hinduism is another major world religion that also originated in India and is a polytheistic religion. Researchers believe Hinduism originated between 2500 to 1500 BCE; however, it is appears to have become a dominant faith in Southeast Asia during the fourth century CE. During the early twenty-first century, an estimated 80 percent of India's population practiced Hinduism. Hindu religious tradition emphasizes doctrine, practice, society, story, and devotion. Hindu doctrine maintains there is a relationship between the divine and the world, acknowledges the disparity between world preserving ideals and a flawed world, and addresses the destiny of an individual as opposed to their ties to family and society. Hindu practice honors a deity, especially through the giving and sharing of food. Hindu society separates society into four ideal castes: Brahmans (priests), Kshatriyas (warriors and nobles), Vaishyas (commoners), and Shudras (servants). Hindu stories pass along traditions that occurred between the gods and humans over a two-millennial period. Hindu devotion is the last strand of Hindu belief that emphasizes devotion to a loving god. Karma describes the principle of cause and effect, also known as fate.

Karma and reincarnation are two of the major tenets of Hinduism. Hindus believe that actions and reactions, through karma, govern consciousness. Hindus also believe that all souls reincarnate, going from body to body while spiritually evolving over time. Hindu scriptures emphasize nonviolence as a path to spirituality. According to the Yajur Veda, a book of Hindu prayers, "You must not use your God-given body for killing God's creatures, whether they be human, animals, or whatever" (12.32). Mahatma Gandhi, an Indian social activist who lived from 1869 to 1948, declared, "The greatness of a nation and its moral progress can be measured by the way in which its animals are treated." Hindus believe consuming an animal causes bad karma, or negative consequences, for the person as a consequence of ill treatment of others. While the practice of vegetarianism is encouraged for all Hindus, it still is not a requirement of the faith. The *Manu-smriti*, a book of Hindu laws, states, "There is no sin in eating meat . . . but abstention brings great rewards" (5:56). It is estimated, based on a 2004 census of Hindus in India, that 25 percent of the Indian population is vegetarian. Early Hinduism involved animal sacrifices, and some sects continue to follow this practice today. But the concept of reincarnation holds that every life on earth, including insects and animals, is reborn into the next life. It is thought that a human who lives a bad life is reborn into a lower caste or as an animal. Thus, to kill or eat an animal is bad karma, and vegetarian diets should be followed.

Jainism is commonly believed to have originated in eastern India during the seventh to fifth centuries BCE. It is considered be a polytheistic religion because Jainism believes all souls are divine. Derived from the Sanskrit verb "to conquer," Jainism believes that complete perfection and purification of the soul is paramount by overcoming the bodily senses.

Jain tenets adhere to ahimsa (nonviolence), *aparigraha* (nonacquisition), *asteya* (respect for other beings), and *satya* (truth). Following the religious principles of Jainism leads to ultimate salvation. Jainists believe that karmas, which they describe as bits of material that are generated by a person's actions, attach themselves to the soul and are passed from person to person as they are reborn. This in turn prohibits freedom of the soul. They also believe that it is wrong to kill or harm any living thing. Compassion for all life, human and nonhuman, is a basic tenet of Jainism. Cows are treated as members of the family because of the belief of reincarnation. Thus in Jainism, vegetarian diets are mandatory for those who follow the faith as a way to earn meritorious rebirth that will bring them closer to a pure state. While milk and milk products and eggs are not prohibited in the diet, they are eliminated during important Jain religious celebrations. Honey is forbidden because of the belief harvesting is harmful to bees. Potatoes and other root vegetables are forbidden because harvesting may kill insects and bacteria that exist in the plant.

Taoism, a nontheistic religion, is a religion that evolved in China during the fourth to third centuries BCE. Tao is considered the essential energy of life, and the concepts of Yin and Yang are core philosophies of Tao. Yin and Yang represent a balance of positive and negative energies within the universe, such as up and down, masculine and feminine, good and bad, or darkness and light. Yin and Yang also characterize the opposites that occur naturally throughout life that then provides the energy of Tao. The religion of Taoism believes all of nature is sacred. Meat is considered to be a corrupting influence within Chinese medicine practice, and Taoism teaches meat is too yang, or aggressive, thus negatively impacting the environment. The *Tao Te Ching*, the central text and guide credited to founder Lao-tzu, teaches that simplicity and the protection of nature from overuse and pollution promotes a peaceful life. Taoism encourages following a vegetarian diet and abstaining from meat. However, it does not restrict Taoists from eating meat if they so choose. The typical Taoist diet emphasizes eating foods that are "natural" and are not highly processed or contain human-made preservatives or additives. Food choices are to come primarily from vegetables and fruits. Minimal amounts of meat or fish, poultry, or game birds are allowed. Early Taoist diets prohibited grains because it was thought that grains fed worms living in the gastrointestinal tract that shortened the life of an individual. Modern Taoists include whole grains in their daily diet.

Judaism, Christianity, and Islam are the major religions found outside of Asian countries. Judaism is considered the oldest monotheistic religion in the world, and followers believe there is only one God. It is thought to have originated over 3,500 years ago in the Middle East. The Torah contains the first five books of Hebrew scriptures, which are considered the recorded laws of God. The principles of Jewish faith are stated in the Tanakh (the written Torah, including more than the first five books) and the oral Torah (Talmud). It is generally accepted that the first people of the earth were vegetarians based on the scripture verses in the first book of the Torah. The Book of Bereishit, also known as Genesis, chapter 1, verses 29 and 30, states: "And God said, "Behold, I have given you every seed bearing herb, which is upon the surface of the entire earth, and every tree that has seed bearing fruit; it will be yours for food. And to all the beasts of the earth and to all the fowl of the heavens, and to everything that moves upon the earth, in which there is a living spirit, every green herb to eat, and it was so." However, Genesis, chapter 9, verse 3, relates that God told Noah, after the flood, "Every moving thing that lives shall be yours to eat; like the green vegetation, I have given you everything," indicating that animals later became an approved food source due to human weakness.

Judaism has strict dietary laws, known as kosher laws, that its follow-ers must adhere to. Judaism also forbids inflicting unnecessary pain on animals, and a trained religious individual, called a schochet, must per-form the method of animal slaughter. Only animals that have a cloven hoof and chew cud, such as cattle, sheep, and goats, may be eaten. Pigs are forbidden. Fish, poultry, pigeons, and fowl are allowed, but shellfish is prohibited. Eggs are allowed, but only from kosher animals that do not eat any feed that includes animal blood. Eggs and dairy are allowed but may not be eaten together with meat or poultry or fowl. Dairy and eggs may be eaten with fish. Other foods are banned during special holidays in the Jewish faith, such as Passover. Rabbi Shlomo Riskin, an Orthodox Israeli rabbi, states: "The dietary laws are intended to teach us compassion and lead us gently to vegetarianism."

Christianity, another major monotheistic religion, began as a separate denomination of Judaism. The Jewish Tanakh foretells the coming of the Mashiach, or Messiah, who will be anointed as King in the End of Days. The End of Days marks a time of great political and societal unrest, wars, and suffering. The Messiah will come to restore everlasting peace and salvation, establishing Judaism as the law of the land. Christians believe that the Messiah already came in the person of Jesus of Nazareth. Jesus, a Jewish rabbi born around 5–4 BCE, is claimed to have fulfilled all prophe-cies in the Tanakh describing the Messiah. As described in the Bible, Jesus was crucified around 26–36 CE by the Romans as the King of the Jews and resurrected on the third day. He spent time with his followers before ascending to Heaven and is to return at the End of Days.

Like Judaism, Christianity prohibits cruelty to animals. Jesus taught his followers to love and have compassion and mercy for all others. The Bible is the Christian text that believers follow. It is comprised of the Old Testament and New Testament. The Old Testament books are similar to those found in the Jewish Tanakh. Genesis, chapter 1, verses 29 and 30, (NIV) states: "Then God said, 'I give you every seed-bearing plant on the face of the whole earth and every tree that has fruit with seed in it. They will be yours for food. And to all the beasts of the earth and all the birds in the sky and all the creatures that move along the ground—everything that has the breath of life in it—I give every green plant for food. And it was so.'" As in Judaism, these verses are cited to indicate that early humans were meant to be vegetarians. But as in the Tanakh, animal foods were approved as food after the flood when God told Noah in Genesis, chapter 9, verse 3, (NIV): "Everything that lives and moves about will be food for you. Just as I gave you the green plants, I now give you everything." While the Old Testament laws governed what foods were acceptable to eat or prohibited for believers, the New Testament, written by the followers of Jesus, shifted away from the strict kosher laws of the Old Testament and Tanakh.

The Apostle Paul wrote in Romans, chapter 14, verses 2 and 3: "One person's faith allows them to eat anything, but another, whose faith is weak, eats only vegetables. The one who eats everything must not treat with contempt the one who does not, and the one who does not eat everything must not judge the one who does, for God has accepted them." Verse 6 states: "Whoever regards one day as special does so to the Lord. Whoever eats meat does so to the Lord, for they give thanks to God; and whoever abstains does so to the Lord and gives thanks to God." These Bible verses imply that plant-based diets are not a central tenet required for the faithful. But the care of and kindness toward animals is taught, as seen in Proverbs, chapter 12, verse 10, (NIV), which states: "The righteous care for the needs of their animals, but the kindest acts of the wicked are cruel." Many Christians choose to follow plant-based diets because of their concern over the humane treatment of animals. Animal cruelty is inconsistent with Christian beliefs. Some Christians believe that Jesus was a vegetarian. But New Testament scriptures do not validate this theory. Luke, chapter 24, verses 42 and 43, (NIV) states: "They gave him (Jesus) a piece of broiled fish, and he took it and ate it in their presence." It is also well known that Jesus followed rabbinic law and the Torah, eating the yearly Passover lamb.

One other large religious group, Islam, does have a diet rich in plant-based foods but does not require an animal-free diet. In fact, animal sacrifice is an important tenet of the Islamic faith, although the Holy Qur'an does encourage kindness to animals and strict rules are to be followed for animal slaughter. During Eid al Adha, an important Muslim celebration, it is reported that an estimated 100 million animals are ritually slaughtered over a 48-hour time period. While following a vegetarian or vegan diet is considered a deviation from the faith for many Muslims, the Vegan Muslim Initiative estimates an increasing number of Muslims are turning toward veganism.

Aside from religious beliefs, different cultures view plant-based diets differently. In general, Western cultures have a much different opinion of vegetarianism and veganism when compared to eastern cultures. South Asian cultures, while rooted in religious beliefs, have a long history of following plant-based diets. Africa, Israel, Lebanon, Turkey, and other Arab countries include plant-based foods as the main staple of their meal plan citing religious reasons as well as the fact that they live in the Fertile Crescent, which is abundant in agriculture. Although meat and other animal proteins are not excluded from their diet, meatless meals are popular in these countries, and meat consumption is lower when compared to westernized countries. The main staple of many westernized countries is meat due to agricultural practices and farming technology that has evolved over time.

Plant-Based Diets and Health

8. What are the potential health benefits of plant-based diets?

Numerous research studies point to the fact that plant-based diets appear to be highly effective in the treatment and management of many chronic illnesses, particularly high blood pressure, cardiovascular disease, diabetes, and obesity. Research studies are frequently used to study specific health related subjects. There are many different study designs used to collect data. The type of study method selected depends upon the goals and subject of the study. However, it can be very difficult to establish the direct cause for a chronic illness due to the fact chronic illnesses develop over a long period of time and can be attributed to many variables besides diet. But a large number of studies do support a direct correlation between health and diet habits. Some of the following studies explore this diet and health connection.

In 2013, physicians Philip Tuso, Mohamed Ismail, and Benjamin Ha and registered dietitian Carole Bartolotto reviewed published studies evaluating the impact plant-based diets have on rates of diabetes, heart disease, longevity, and weight loss due to the fact that rates of cardiovascular disease, diabetes, hypertension, and obesity were increasing again after a period of decline in America. It is well known that eating a diet high in red meat increases rates for all-cause mortalities. The researchers defined plant-based diets as a diet rich in nutrient dense whole, plant-based foods with minimal processed foods, dairy, meat, and eggs. When they looked at cardiovascular disease studies, they found plant-based diets had a positive impact on the prevention and reversal of heart disease as well as the lowering of blood pressure. Although many of the studies analyzed diets that included minimal amounts of animal foods, such as the Mediterranean diet, one study found ischemic heart disease deaths were reduced by 24 percent in vegetarians when compared to nonvegetarians. A 73 percent decrease in heart attacks and strokes and 70 percent decrease for all-cause mortality was also seen in those who followed a Mediterranean diet. Comprehensive lifestyle changes and a plant-based meal plan, even with the inclusion of small amounts of animal foods, are found to reduce the overall risk for cardiovascular diseases and mortality. However, the inclusion of some animal foods in the diet is a point of controversy among some physicians. Dr. Dean Ornish, a researcher and cardiologist who founded the Preventive Medicine Research Institute in California, advocates no more than two servings a day of low-fat dairy and egg whites as acceptable inclusions in the diet for reversing heart disease. In contrast, Dr. Caldwell Esselstyn, a specialist in cardiovascular disease at the Cleveland Clinic Wellness Institute, recommends avoiding all animal-based foods as well as soybeans and nuts if an individual has severe coronary artery disease.

In studies that evaluated diabetes risk, Tuso and his colleagues found vegetarians reduced their risk for diabetes by 50 percent. Nonvegetarians were noted to be 74 percent more likely to develop diabetes when followed over a 17-year period of time. Following a low-fat plant-based diet was also found to have additional health benefits for diabetics. Forty-three percent of diabetics who ate a low-fat vegan diet were able to reduce their medication when compared to 26 percent of diabetics who followed the American Diabetes Association diabetic diet. The American Diabetes Association diabetic diet emphasizes a diet mainly of vegetables, low sugar fruits, legumes, whole grains, healthy fats, low-fat dairy, and lean meats, chicken, and fish. Carbohydrate choices are limited in amount, and processed foods and sugars are eliminated.

Tuso's review also looked at 87 studies correlating a vegetarian or vegan diet with weight loss. The majority of studies found vegetarian or vegan meal plans were highly effective for weight loss, independent of exercise. In 2015, the results of the New DIETs study was published in *Eating Behaviors*. These researchers examined participants who ate vegan, vegetarian, omnivore, pescovegetarian, or semivegetarian diets. Questionnaires and 24-hour diet recalls were used to gather data for analysis of diet impact on health. They found vegans and vegetarians experienced more weight loss than those individuals who included animal foods in their diet. The researchers concluded that diet choices, along with lifestyle choice, were strongly linked to chronic illnesses and obesity.

In 2009, researchers Yang and Beysoun analyzed NHANES data collected from 1999 to 2004. They also found a positive association between meat consumption and obesity. An Oxford study of the European Prospective Investigation into Cancer and Nutrition studied weight gain among omnivores, vegetarians, and vegans in the United Kingdom. A total of 21,966 men and women between the ages of 20 and 69 were first studied from 1994 to 1999 and then reevaluated from 2000 to 2003. Although the Oxford study found small differences in weight gain among meat eaters, fish eaters, vegetarians, or vegans, they still concluded that individuals who ate fewer animal foods had the lowest total amount of weight gain over time. Overall, studies find overwhelming evidence that those who eat a plant-based diet have lower rates of diabetes, heart disease, high blood pressure, and obesity.

9. What are the potential negative health consequences of following a plant-based diet?

Plant-based diets are often assumed to be the best way to eat for good health. However, this isn't always a correct assumption. As seen in Question 8, there is evidence that points to positive health benefits from following a plant-based diet. But planning and maintaining the proper balance of nutritionally adequate foods daily is critically important for good health. When animal foods are eliminated from the diet, malnutrition can occur if the right balance of foods are not selected or nutrients supplemented properly. Deficiencies of vitamin B_{12}, vitamin D, calcium, iron, omega-3 fatty acids, riboflavin, and zinc are most commonly found in vegans when attention is not paid to proper diet planning. Deficiencies of vitamin B_{12} can occur suddenly or gradually and be confused with other causes. Symptoms of a vitamin B_{12} deficiency include anemia, balance difficulties, fatigue, cognitive difficulties or memory loss, swollen and inflamed tongue, and weakness. A vitamin D deficiency can cause a loss of bone density contributing to osteoporosis, rickets, and fractures. Symptoms of a calcium deficiency can cause abdominal cramps, loss of bone density, spasms of the hands and feet, muscle cramps, osteoporosis, and rickets. Iodine deficiencies can cause hypothyroidism and contribute to birth defects in an unborn child. Iron deficiencies can cause anemia, poor appetite, extreme fatigue, chest pain, shortness of breath, headache, cold hands or feet, brittle nails, pica, and weakness. Deficiency of omega-3 fatty acids can cause dermatitis or rough and scaly skin. Zinc deficiencies can slow growth in infants and children, delay sexual development in teens, and cause impotence in adult males, loss of appetite, diarrhea, hair loss, eye and skin sores, and weight loss. Nutrient deficiencies are further discussed further in Question 18.

Some vegans and vegetarians also gain weight when following a plant-based diet. This is often the result of selecting highly processed carbohydrate foods that are high in fat and sugar while neglecting to eat adequate plant-based protein and vegetables. Conversely, some vegans and vegetarians lose weight or have difficulty maintaining a normal weight because they choose to eat large amounts of vegetables and fruit and do not eat enough protein, complex carbohydrates, or fat. This results in eating too few calories, which can also lead to negative health consequences and is the result of a poorly planned diet.

Plant-based diets are also high in dietary fiber, which can cause gastrointestinal intolerance when the total amount of daily fiber is not started slowly and gradually increased to optimal levels. The average animal-based diet is estimated to provide 15–17 grams of fiber per day. One benefit of plant-based diet is the high fiber content of plants. Fiber is the substance found in the outer layers of grains or plants that are not digested in the small and large intestines. There are two types of fiber: soluble and insoluble. Soluble fiber is made of carbohydrates and dissolves in water and is found in barley, fruit, legumes, and oats. Insoluble fiber is found in the cell walls of plants and does not dissolve in water. It is found in wheat bran, rye, and other grains. The Academy of Nutrition and Dietetics recommends 25 grams of fiber per day for women, 28 grams of fiber for pregnant and lactating women, and 38 grams of fiber per day for men. Adults aged 50 or older are advised to eat less fiber: 21 grams per day for women and 28 grams of fiber per day for men. Eating a diet that has a minimum recommended daily amount of 20–25 grams is found to decrease symptoms of constipation, diarrhea, fecal incontinence, and hemorrhoids and may also reduce the risk for cardiovascular disease, diabetes, and stroke. It can also reduce symptoms of irritable bowel disease or diverticulosis. However, for some people increased amounts of dietary fiber can make symptoms worse, signifying gastrointestinal intolerance that manifests as bloating, constipation, diarrhea, passing of gas, or intestinal pain. Extreme cases may develop a small bowel obstruction, which often requires surgical repair.

Another aspect often overlooked is the fact that plants have a defense system that protects the plant from predators that might eat them and put the plant species at risk for extinction. Plants have naturally occurring phytochemicals, also called antinutrients, which are biologically active compounds. These antinutrients discourage animals, fungi, insects, and humans from eating them because they often have a bitter taste or cause gastrointestinal upset. Some of these compounds can also be toxic with the more valuable parts of a plant more toxic than the rest of the plant. For example, seeds are critical for the survival of a plant species. Grains are considered the seeds of corn, oats, rice, and wheat. Hazelnuts, pecans, and walnuts are the seeds of trees. Legumes, such as chickpeas, lentils, peas, peanuts, and soybeans, are seeds of beans. There are two types of seeds: protected and naked. Protected seeds are found in a protective shell, like nuts, and naked seeds are exposed, like those found in tomatoes and wheat. Naked seeds are more toxic because they are exposed. This exposure results in naked seeds containing chemical compounds that can make them bitter to taste and may also cause intestinal lining damage to whoever eats them. This in turn causes inflammation and malabsorption of nutrients and gastrointestinal distress that usually ensures the animal will avoid eating them in the future. This then protects the plants' chances for survival.

Some of these toxins are thought to be the root cause of allergies, autoimmune diseases, food sensitivities, and other chronic illnesses in humans who cannot tolerate them. For example, walnuts contain phytic acid that can bind itself to calcium, iron, magnesium, phosphorus, and zinc. When phytic acid binds these essential minerals, they are not absorbed in the gastrointestinal tract, and this could contribute to malnutrition. Malnutrition is the improper balance of essential vitamins and minerals in the daily diet, leading to illness and disease. Unlike cows and sheep, which have bacteria in their gastrointestinal tract to breakdown phytates, humans are not designed to eat only plants and thus do not have these bacteria in their gastrointestinal tract. Because of this, if walnuts are overconsumed nutritional deficiencies can occur.

Phytic acid also interferes with absorption of nonheme iron found in plants. When meat, which is a rich source of iron, is eliminated from the diet anemia can occur. Anemia is a disease in which blood does not contain enough healthy red blood cells or hemoglobin. Hemoglobin, a crucial component of red blood cells, binds with oxygen. When hemoglobin levels are too low, individual cells cannot get enough oxygen, leading to severe fatigue. There are over 400 different types of anemia, and iron is a critical component of hemoglobin. There are two different forms of iron found in food: heme and nonheme. Heme iron is found only in fish, meat, poultry, and seafood. Nonheme iron is found in plant foods, such as beans, dairy, eggs, fruits, grain, nuts, seeds, and vegetables. Studies find that vegetarians have higher incidences of anemia even though they consume more iron from plant sources than meat eaters. One study found 40 percent of vegan women were deficient in iron despite eating the minimally recommended amount of iron daily.

Other examples of these antinutrients are enzyme inhibitors, glycoalkaloids, glucosinolate, lectins, myrosinase, oxalates, saponins, and sulforaphane. Soybeans have enzyme inhibitors that can inflame the gastrointestinal tract and interfere with protein digestion. Soybeans also have saponins, which protect the plant from microbes and fungi. Saponins have been linked to autoimmune diseases, gut inflammation, and leaky gut in humans. Wheat has lectin, which is a natural insecticide, and resistant to human digestion. Lectins have been associated with intestinal inflammation, leaky gut, malabsorption, and interference with starch digestion. Potatoes contain glycoalkaloids, which are neurotoxins that overstimulate the nervous system and can cause convulsions, paralysis, and, in extreme cases, death. One glycoalkaloid, solanine, is found in nightshade vegetables (eggplants, peppers, potatoes, and tomatoes), and the maximum legal limit regulated by the United States government can be no more than 200 mg/kg of potatoes. Cruciferous vegetables, such as broccoli, have glucosinolate and myrosinase and sulforaphane, all recognized to have anticancer properties. However, eating too much of these chemicals in the diet can have negative effects on thyroid health and the gastrointestinal system. Oxalates are another protective chemical found in some plants such as spinach. Too much oxalate in the diet binds calcium and may cause kidney disease, malabsorption of calcium and iron, and is sometimes fatal. Oxalates are also found in beans, berries, chocolate, cruciferous vegetables, kale, okra, potatoes, most nuts, sesame and poppy seeds, soy, sweet potatoes, and swiss chard. Various fruits have salicylates, cyanogenic glycosides, flavonoids, photosensitizers, and tannins that all can have negative impacts on health when overconsumed. Although these antinutrients can result in negative health consequences, a plant-based diet can be safely consumed when properly planned, when plant foods are prepared correctly, and when plant foods are eaten in moderation.

Salicylates are another compound that can be problematic for someone eating a plant-based diet. A salicylate intolerance occurs when the immune system overreacts to normal amounts of salicylates found in foods. Salicylates are derivatives of salicylic acid. Salicylic acid occurs naturally in plants and is part of a plants immune system that it to defend against bacteria, fungi, insects, and disease. Most fruits and vegetables, spices, herbs, flavor additives, and tea have naturally occurring salicylates, although some processed foods may have them added. Mint flavors, tomato sauce, berries, processed foods, and citrus fruits have the highest levels of salicylates.

Another aspect of plant-based diets often overlooked is its tie to eating disorders. Eating disorders are detrimental to health and are complex psychological, physiological, and social diseases that are not easily treated and have a poor treatment success rate. At least 30 million people are estimated to have some form of eating disorder in the United States, according to the National Association of Anorexia Nervosa and Associated Disorders (ANAD). Eating disorders also have the highest mortality rate of any mental illness. The most well-studied eating disorder, anorexia nervosa, occurs when a person refuses to eat in an obsessive desire to lose weight. Because many people are not well informed about what a vegetarian or vegan diet entails, many anorexics often use the excuse of following a plant-based diet to hide their illness. Still others become obsessed with eliminating animal foods from their diet, resulting in orthorexia. Orthorexia is another eating disorder that is defined as a change in eating habits that becomes an obsession with eating only "healthy foods." A 2012 study by Bardone-Cone and colleagues found that 61 percent of eating disorder patients believed there was a relationship between their choosing a vegetarian diet and their eating disorder. These researchers also found that about 50 percent of anorexia nervosa patients claimed to follow a vegetarian diet and were the least likely to be successful with treatment. However, they also found that most eating disorder patients were eating a vegetarian diet for at least one year prior to their diagnosis. They concluded that people who are predisposed to eating disorders were more likely to choose a vegetarian meal plan.

Another unexpected downside of vegetarianism is the connection between eating a vegetarian diet and depression. Hal Herzog, PhD, investigated this connection and summarized his findings in *Psychology Today*. Looking at 11 peer-reviewed studies, he found that the majority of vegetarians and semivegetarians had higher rates of depression than nonvegetarians. The exact reason for this is unclear. One theory is that meat contains the amino acid tryptophan, which is a precursor for the neurotransmitter serotonin. Serotonin is believed to play a critical role in the prevention of anxiety and depression. It is speculated that when brain serotonin levels are decreased, depression and anxiety risk is increased. Potential vitamin B_{12}, vitamin A, vitamin D, iron, and zinc deficiencies also play a role in depression and anxiety risk. It is also speculated that brain chemistry and microbiome changes from eating a plant-based diet may have an impact on risk for depression and anxiety.

10. Do genetics influence whether or not a plant-based diet is healthy for an individual?

Every human is born with a set of genes that determines what he or she looks like and how predisposed they are to illnesses and chronic disease. Genes are made of deoxyribonucleic acid (DNA), which is like a blueprint or set of instructions that individual body cells read and follow to function properly. DNA is a double strand of genetic information shaped like a ladder whose structure is made of molecules, called bases, known as adenine (A), thymine (T), guanine (G), and cytosine (C). Ribonucleic acid (RNA) is similar to DNA but is a single strand of genetic information that carries messages from DNA used to synthesize proteins and transport these proteins into the areas where they are needed in the cells. DNA contains all the genetic information necessary for an organism to live. Every person inherits two copies of this DNA "alphabet," one from each parent. Approximately 99 percent of genes are the same for everyone in the world. But slight variations in the remaining 1 percent of genes contain the small differences that give individuals their unique physical attributes, distinguishing them from everyone else.

In general, the DNA base pairs A and T always pair together, and the G base always pairs up with the C base. Because every single cell in the body contains a complete set of DNA instructions, DNA is constantly being copied as new cells replace old ones. A single nucleotide polymorphism (SNP), or allele, is a copying error that can occur during this process, pairing bases differently from the rule. For instance, A may pair up with C instead of T as the result of a copying error. When the bases pair incorrectly, genetic susceptibility for diseases or other conditions is increased. But this does not mean an individual will definitely develop a disease. Other factors, such as environment, diet, or lifestyle choices, also affect genes or gene SNP combinations and can either "turn on" a susceptible gene, causing a chronic disease or immune system malfunction, or "turn off" the gene to reduce the risk for a disease. In 2001, the Human Genome Project announced the successful mapping of 90 percent of the genome sequence of the 3 billion base-pairs of the human genome. Published in the journal *Nature* in February 2001, this only began our understanding of how genes influence disease and chronic illness in humans.

"Genetics" and "genomics" are the terms used to define the constantly evolving science of genes and their influence on health. The Merriam-Webster dictionary defines "genetics" as "a specific sequence of nucleotides in DNA or RNA that is located usually on a chromosome and that is the functional unit of inheritance controlling the transmission and expression of one or more traits by specifying the structure of a particular polypeptide and especially a protein or controlling the function of other genetic material." The Merriam-Webster dictionary further defines "genomics" as "a branch of biotechnology concerned with applying techniques of genetics and molecular biology to the genetic mapping and DNA sequencing of sets of genes or the complete genomes of selected organisms, with organizing the results in databases, and with applications of the data (as in medicine or biology)." Genomics is further distinguished into epigenetics, which is the science of changes that occur to inherited genes as the result of environmental factors. These changes occur naturally all through the lifecycle but do not change the underlying DNA structure of the gene. Gene combinations act like recipes, which cells read and follow to function properly. Known as heritable changes, gene expression (the recipe) can be influenced by environment, lifestyle, and the foods we eat. These heritable changes in turn can also cause errors in the gene "recipe," possibly causing chronic diseases or immune system malfunctions.

Studies investigating human gene response to plant-based diets are still in their infancy. To date, studies investigating the relationship between diet and genes have explored their impact on cancer, individual nutrient utilization, and blood types. Researchers at Cornell University discovered that populations with a history of plant-based diets had genetic differences from those who included animal foods in their diet. In 2016, Cornell University researchers, funded by the National Institutes of Health (NIH) and the U.S. Department of Agriculture, investigated long-term genetic changes that could occur in populations that eat a predominantly vegetarian diet. Individuals in Africa, America, Asia, Europe, Greenland, and India were evaluated. They identified populations that appear to have adapted genetically to a predominantly plant-based way of eating by developing "vegetarian alleles." Individuals with these polymorphisms were able to more efficiently process omega-3 and omega-6 fatty acids. Omega-3s and omega-6s are essential fatty acids necessary for good health and are not synthesized by the human body. This means that including essential fatty acids in the daily diet is important to maintain health. Omega-3s are found in fish, flax seeds, some fruits, olive oil, vegetables, and whole grains. Omega-6s are found in beef, many snack and processed foods, nuts, and vegetable oils. Diets in westernized countries tend to have a 15:1 ratio of omega-6s to omega-3s. Because omega-3s have anti-inflammatory properties, diets high in omega-6s are thought to be a cause of high levels of inflammation leading to chronic illnesses in westernized countries, such as heart disease and diabetes. It is generally assumed that the ratio of omega-3s to omega-6s should be eaten in a 1:1 ratio and that the Mediterranean meal plan most closely achieves this goal.

However, this study found that the ratio of essential fatty acids needed by an individual actually varies from person to person, depending on their genes. Thus, choice of the most effective diet for good health must be personalized, rather than following a one-diet-fits-all approach. One example of the impact genes have on diet and health is the FADs gene. Cornell researchers found 70 percent of South Asians, 68 percent of Indians, 53 percent of Africans, 29 percent of East Asians, 17 percent of Europeans, and 18 percent of Americans had the vegetarian allele due to their vegetarian diet habits. They also found the Inuits in Greenland had a "marine allele," showing their adaptation to a seafood rich diet. These vegetarian and marine alleles appear to control the FADS1 and FADS2 enzymes, which are made within the body to convert omega-3s and omega-6s into compounds needed for brain development and inflammation control. Individuals who eat meat and seafood were found to need less of the FADS1 and FADS2 enzymes than those who eat only plant-based diets. However, the genes of those groups who ate mostly a plant-based diet appeared to become modified as an adaptation to that diet, thus allowing those who eat mostly plants to more efficiently convert essential fatty acids in their foods for use in the body. It is interesting to note that individuals who eat plant-based diets often consume more omega-3s than those who eat a meat-based diet, yet they continue to remain at a higher risk for omega-3 deficiencies.

Cancers are caused by a number of different variables, including diet, lifestyle, and environment. In 1981, researchers Richard Doll and Richard Peto estimated genetics affects cancer risk by 2–3 percent. A review of their work in 2015 continues to uphold this estimate and the fact that there are many other factors, besides genetics, that can create a long-term or fatal disease. However, genetics can make some individuals more susceptible to diet, lifestyle, and environmental carcinogens by having the ability to "turn on" cancer genes. Johanna W. Lampe, of the Fred Hutchinson Cancer Research Center, investigated genetic differences and their influence on taste preference, food tolerance, and phytochemical absorption and metabolism in relation to cancer risk when eating a plant-based diet. Lampe's primary goal was to identify cancer-related genes and gene SNPs influenced by diet. She reported her findings in the 2009 *American Journal of Clinical Nutrition*.

Environmental carcinogens and xenobiotics, compounds that also occur naturally or are human-made in the environment, have been linked to increased cancer rates. The human body has detoxification systems that remove these toxic compounds, via the kidneys, intestines, liver, lungs, lymph system, and skin. The detoxification system converts harmful compounds that enter the body to less harmful by-products for removal using biotransformation enzymes during the process of glucuronidation. Glucuronidation is the metabolic reaction the body uses to remove these harmful by-products. Genes and gene SNPs regulate the manufacture of these biotransformation enzymes and has an impact on how well individuals remove toxins from their bodies.

Lampe identified that foods in our daily diet, besides having beneficial nutrients, also include carcinogens and xenobiotics. She also found that while phytochemicals, which are nonnutrient chemical compounds found in many plant-based foods, have a positive effect biologically and usually reduce cancer risk, some gene SNPs can actually negatively affect their positive impact and subsequently increase cancer risk rather than protect against it. For example, Glutathione S-transerases (GSTs), UDP-glucuronosyltransferases (UGTs), and sulfotransferases (SULTs) are enzymes that have the ability to remove carcinogens and other xenobiotics from the body. A gene SNP on any of the pathways that produce these enzymes may have profound implications on how well toxins are removed from the body and potentially increase cancer risk. Thus, while a plant-based diet contains many phytonutrients that protect against cancer, individual gene SNPs may negate their protective effect.

Studies also show that gene SNPs affect how well individuals convert vitamins and minerals in their diet to active forms needed to maintain health. There are a number of vitamins and minerals, supplied by the diet, that are essential for optimal health. Most of these nutrients must undergo an activation process so that the nutrient can be utilized properly. One example involves the BCMO1 gene. Individuals who have a BCMO1 gene SNP do not convert vitamin A to its active form efficiently. Plant foods contain vitamin A precursors, such as beta-carotene. These precursors are converted in the liver and intestine by the enzyme beta-carotene -15,15'-monoxygenase (BCMO1) to the active form of vitamin A, which the body is then able to use in a number of different ways. Animal foods, in contrast, don't require the BCMO1 conversion to the active form because animal foods have the active form of vitamin A already available for use. Individuals with BCMO1 polymorphisms are estimated to have a reduced beta-carotene conversion rate of 69 percent, putting them at risk for a vitamin A deficiency. Vitamin A deficiencies can cause xerophthalmia, otherwise known as night blindness (the inability to see in low light or darkness), blindness, and susceptibility to severe or fatal infections. Those who eat a plant-based diet with no or few animal foods and have the BCMO1 gene have an increased susceptibility for a vitamin A deficiency.

Another example is the amylase-coding gene (AMY1), which manufactures alpha-amylase, found in human saliva and used to digest starch molecules into simple sugars for use as energy in the body. Populations that tend to eat diets high in starch or carbohydrate foods have been found to have more AMY1 genes, and consequently more alpha-amylase in their saliva, than those who eat predominantly high fat and protein diets. This difference in alpha-amylase availability also affects how well blood sugar is regulated, putting those with low amylase production at risk for diabetes and obesity. Individuals who eat a plant-based diet that is high in carbohydrates, and have AMY1 gene variations, are at an increased risk for carbohydrate intolerance, negating the positive impact of a plant-based diet.

Individuals who have a phosphatidylethanolamine-N-methyltransferase (PEMT) gene SNP may also be at risk for choline deficiencies. Choline is an essential nutrient important for metabolism, brain health, neurotransmitter synthesis, lipid transport, and methylation. Choline deficiencies are associated with fatty liver disease, heart disease, neurological disorders, and developmental problems in children. Choline is primarily found in animal foods, such as egg yolks, liver, meat and seafood. Plant foods do have some choline, but at reduced amounts in comparison to animal foods. Choline can be produced within the body, but those with PEMT gene SNPs and who eat a plant-based diet are at an increased risk for a choline deficiency.

One last theory that needs to be discussed due to its popularity among many patients who try alternative medicine treatments is the blood type diet. Dr. Peter J. D'Adamo, a naturopathic physician, developed the blood type diet in 1996. Dr. D'Adamo posits that the genes we inherit from our parents, which in turn determine our blood type, have an effect on how well an individual processes food. He further theorizes that blood type can have a positive or negative long-term impact on overall health. In 2013, researchers Leila Cusack, Emmy DeBuck, Veerle Compernolle, and Philippe Vandekerckhove reviewed published studies related to blood type diets. Reported in *the American Journal of Clinical Nutrition*, the researchers concluded that there was no evidence supporting health benefits from eating a diet tailored specifically to blood type.

11. What impact do plant-based diets have on the gastrointestinal microbiome?

The human gastrointestinal (GI) tract is a very complex system that acts as an interface between humans and their environment. Trillions of microbes, which are a collection of bacteria, viruses, fungi, and other single celled organisms, live on or in humans. While some microbes can be harmful, the majority live in a symbiotic relationship with their host human. This means that both microbes and humans need each other for survival. Microbes are inherited or established at a young age. For example, bifidobacteria are passed to babies as they travel through the birth canal during the birth process. Bifidobacteria are anaerobic bacteria that make up most of the microbes found in the GI tract of all mammals. The majority of human microbes live in the human GI tract, and the genetic material of these microbes is known as the microbiome. The GI tract contains over 3 million genes, and each individual's microbiome is unique.

The microbiome digests food, regulates the immune system, protects against bacteria that cause disease, and produces vitamin K and some B vitamins. The increased importance of the microbiome was discovered during the late 1990s, and we are only just beginning to learn how the microbiome impacts health. Autoimmune diseases, such as diabetes, rheumatoid arthritis, fibromyalgia, multiple sclerosis, and muscular dystrophy, are all linked to imbalances of the microbiome. It is speculated that inheriting the family microbiome, rather than inheriting family DNA, may actually be the cause of many autoimmune diseases common in some families. For instance, obese twins are found to have a lower diversity of bacteria and higher levels of enzymes in their GI microbiome when compared to twins who are lean. This indicates the microbiome of the obese twins is more efficient at digesting food and harvesting calories, causing weight gain and difficulty in losing weight. The Human Microbiome Project (HMP), sponsored by the National Human Genome Research Institute, is a worldwide research initiative that studies the microbiome of humans. As associations are made between the microbiome and susceptibility to infectious diseases and chronic illnesses, the hope is effective therapies for treatment or prevention will be discovered.

The diversity of the microbiome also changes during a human's lifetime. Age, use of antibiotic medications, diet, and environment can all alter the human microbiome. Although there are many variables that can change the microbiome, the foods we eat appears to have the most impact on the alteration of bacterial gastrointestinal diversity. It is estimated that during the average lifetime 60 tons of food passes through the human GI tract. Included with foods are many microorganisms and environmental toxins that threaten GI integrity and health. Taking antibiotic medications is also known to destroy bacterial balance in the GI tract, increasing susceptibility to chronic health problems. Prebiotics and probiotics and diet are increasingly used to restore and improve microbial imbalances.

Prebiotics are nondigestible components found in food that feed microbes in the GI tract. Prebiotics are found in artichokes, bananas, garlic, high fiber grains, onions, soybeans, and vegetables. Probiotics are microbes that keep the gut and host human healthy. Microbes are constantly replaced in the GI tract as they age by new microbes coming from foods that have living strains of bacteria or probiotic supplements. Some examples of foods with living probiotics are kombucha, kimchi, sauerkraut, and yogurt.

Studies find that what we eat can quickly change the diversity of our GI microbiome. Harvard researcher Lawrence David and his colleagues found the microbiome could be changed in three days just by altering the diet. They also learned that animal-based diets increased the abundance of bile-tolerant microbes. Bile is a fluid released by the liver to digest foods high in fats, such as meat. Bile tolerant microbes are able to survive the harsh conditions of digestion and increase in number to assist in digesting a diet high in fat. Changes in the microbiome altered by animal-based diets were linked with increased inflammation in the GI tract, which are theorized to contribute to inflammatory bowel diseases.

Eating a plant-based diet appears to positively impact patients with chronic illnesses or who struggle with weight gain. The ratio of firmicutes and bacteroidetes within the GI tract appears to play a significant role in weight management. The most abundant quantities and strains of bacteria that live in the GI tract are classified as bacteroidetes and firmicutes. Researchers studying obese mice found they had a higher ratio of firmicutes to bacteroidetes when compared to lean mice. Firmicute bacteria are very efficient at extracting energy from food when compared to bacteroidetes. This means that a higher firmicute to bacteroidete ratio will increase food conversion to energy to be used or stored as body fat. High fiber diets that are low in fat, sugar, and processed carbohydrates appear to increase bacteroidetes and reduce firmicutes, possibly helping with weight loss efforts. M. S. Kim and colleagues studied obese subjects with adult onset diabetes or hypertension. The study subjects were put on a strict vegetarian diet for one month. All study subjects showed a decrease in firmicutes and an increase in bacteroidetes with subsequent improvements in GI inflammation, lowered cholesterol, triglyceride, and blood sugar levels, as well as weight loss.

R. Peltonen and colleagues studied rheumatoid arthritis patients who traditionally ate a meat-based diet. All study subjects were put on a vegan diet for one year. Significant changes in the microbiome were found in those patients who were compliant with the diet. In a subsequent study, rheumatoid arthritis patients were divided into one group that ate a raw vegan diet and a second group who ate an omnivore diet. The study found the vegan group experienced improvement in symptoms when compared to meat eaters, confirming a connection between the microbiome, a vegan diet, and symptoms for rheumatoid arthritis patients.

R. A. Koeth studied the influence diets have on the microbiome and cardiovascular disease. Vegans, vegetarians, and omnivores were studied over a one-year period. L-carnitine is a dietary derivative of amino acids, found in protein foods. When L-carnitine is digested, trimethlyamine-N-oxide (TMAO) is produced. High levels of TMAO are associated with the promotion of atherosclerosis, which causes increased deposits of fatty plagues on blood artery walls that can cause a heart attack of stroke. The microbiome of vegans and vegetarians showed a different bacterial balance from meat eaters that produced lower amounts of TMAO than the meat eaters, thus reducing their cardiovascular risk.

12. What is the China study, and how does it relate to plant-based diets?

During the early 1970s, the premier of China, Zhou Enlai, was diagnosed with cancer. The premier's illness launched a governmental effort to collect health information about the health status of the Chinese people. This nationwide effort, studying more than 2,400 counties and 880 million citizens, found that different types of cancers varied geographically throughout China. This was of particular interest to researchers because, unlike many westernized countries, the Chinese population is similar in genetic background, with 87 percent of the population belonging to one ethnic group. Researchers concluded that genetics had little impact on cancer incidence and environmental and lifestyle factors likely contributed to the difference in the types and frequency of cancers from county to county.

The data collected by Chinese researchers was summarized in the *Atlas of Cancer Mortality in the People's Republic of China*. Nine types of cancer were found to be common in China: breast, cervix, colon and rectum, esophagus, leukemia, liver, lung, nasopharynx, and stomach. The *Cancer Atlas* pinpointed cancers by county, finding some counties had cancer rates 100 times greater than other counties. These findings attracted interest among the international research community because there was a significant difference in cancer incidence when compared to frequency of cancer in the United States, where cancer rates vary only by 2–3 percent from area to area. The *Cancer Atlas* findings lead to the creation of the

China Project. Researcher T. Colin Campbell, a nutritional biochemist who studied at Cornell University, partnered with researchers at Oxford University and the Chinese Academy of Preventive Medicine in the early 1980s to study the risk for diseases when compared to lifestyle and environment in what has become known as the China study or China Project.

The China study is one of the most extensive nutrition studies ever undertaken that investigates the long-term effects of nutrition and diet habits on human health. The Chinese people were unique because they represented a population that tends to live in the same area while also eating the same unique diet during their entire lifetime. In addition to the original goal of the China study, study results also presented researchers with a unique chance to compare health differences between societies that eat plant-based diets and westernized populations that eat a predominantly animal-based diet.

The Chinese diet is predominantly low in fat and high in dietary fiber and plant foods. The China Project collected data on 367 different variables to determine lifestyle differences among the Chinese population and disease-specific mortality rates. In addition to cancer, frequency of chronic lung disease, ischemic heart disease, and stroke was also studied. Researchers studied an extensive number of individuals over two time periods. From 1983 to 1984, 65 counties in rural China were studied. Within each of these counties, two villages and 50 families were randomly chosen. A total of 6,500 adults, 50 percent women and 50 percent men, were analyzed for diet, lifestyle choices, chronic illnesses, and mortality. Blood, urine, and food samples were collected along with three-day diet records, family interviews, and questionnaires. The same counties and adults were resurveyed from 1989 to 1990; however, 30 new counties in mainland China and Taiwan and 20 new families per county were added. In total, 69 counties and 10,200 adults were studied during the second study period.

The data was then analyzed in an attempt to determine why citizens succumbed to specific diseases. It must be kept in mind that reasons for mortality are not always clearly understood. For instance, smoking habits of men and coal smoke pollution in China are known contributors in the development of many fatal diseases in the Chinese people. But researchers surmised dietary habits were also a major contributing factor due to the fact that westernized countries, which eat more animal foods, had higher rates of disease specific mortality when compared to China. Thus, the China study researchers focused on diet and lifestyle factors that were linked to health outcomes.

In general, researchers find that many chronic illnesses are caused by affluence, which is also closely linked to dietary habits. Diseases most common in affluent societies are cancers (childhood brain, colon, leukemia, liver, and stomach), diabetes, and coronary heart disease. Common diseases of poverty are pneumonia, intestinal obstruction, peptic ulcer, digestive diseases, pulmonary tuberculosis, parasitic infections, rheumatic heart disease, metabolic and endocrine diseases, and pregnancy complications. The China study found that certain diseases clustered together in specific geographic locations, implying a shared cause.

Specific biomarkers, which are substances found in blood that are measurable and indicate the status of the variable being looked at, were evaluated. The researchers found a strong connection between cancer and heart disease and the biomarker blood cholesterol. Cholesterol is a fatty substance made by the liver that is essential for making hormones and necessary for various biochemical reactions within the body. Cholesterol is manufactured within the body but is also found in many animal foods. It has long been assumed in Western cultures that a healthy level of blood cholesterol should range between 125 and 200 mg/dl. Americans have an average cholesterol level of 215 mg/dl. Elevated cholesterol levels over 240 are positively associated with heart disease and cardiac deaths. In Western countries a diet low in saturated fat and cholesterol, sugar, and processed foods along with regular exercise is recommended to keep cholesterol levels low. The American Heart Association in the United States recommends eating foods low in saturated fats, with an emphasis on a heart healthy diet that is high in whole grains, fiber, fish, low-fat dairy, fruits, fish, legumes, nuts, vegetable oils, poultry, and vegetables. Red meat, fried and processed foods, and sugars are discouraged.

The China study found that cholesterol levels decreased significantly when a plant-based diet was eaten in comparison to the recommended low-fat animal-based diet in the United States. China study researchers concluded that animal-based protein appears to increase blood cholesterol levels by a greater amount than saturated fats or cholesterol from foods. The average American consumes 70 grams of animal protein per day compared to the Chinese, who eat an average of 7 grams of animal protein per day. American men with elevated cholesterol levels have a death rate from heart disease 17 times greater than men in rural China. Coronary heart disease rates in the southwestern Chinese provinces were extremely low, with no deaths from heart disease before the age of 64 among 246,000 men and 181,000 women in these provinces.

While elevated blood cholesterol levels in Western countries are associated with heart disease, they have not been traditionally associated with cancer risk. The China study data showed that total fat intake, mainly from animal sources, had a positive correlation to cancer risk. The Chinese people were found to have cholesterol levels that ranged between 80 and 174 mg/dl, with an average cholesterol level of 127 mg/dl. Study results showed that as blood cholesterol levels decreased from 170 mg/dl to 90 mg/dl, cancers of the brain, blood (leukemia), breast, colon, esophagus, liver, lung, rectum, and stomach also decreased.

In 1982, the National Academy of Sciences in the United States recommended that the maximum amount of dietary fat eaten in the daily diet should be no more than 30 percent of total calories. This recommendation was established using international studies that showed an increased risk for breast and large bowel cancer, as well as heart disease, if the amount of dietary fat consumed was greater than 30 percent of total calories. Eating a diet that is no more than 30 percent of calories from fat, no matter the source, is considered a low-fat diet in the United States. Data from the China study found that on average fat comprised 14.5 percent of calories eaten in China. In comparison, the average fat intake for Americans is over 36 percent of calories. However, fat in the food in the Chinese diet is mostly from animal fat, whereas dietary fat in America, besides animal fat, also includes saturated fat from processed plant foods, such as potato chips and French fries. The differences in fat eaten among the Chinese and Americans highlighted the difference upon health between a plant-based diet and an animal-based diet.

Results from the China Study also showed that lowering intake of dietary fat from 24 percent to 6 percent was associated with a lower risk for breast cancer. There are many other risk factors that contribute to breast cancer, such as early age of menstruation, high blood cholesterol, late menopause, and prolonged exposure to female hormones. But high fat diets are associated with early age of menstruation and thus prolonged exposure to female hormones. In China, the average age of menstruation is 17 versus 11 years in the United States, and the age of menopause in the United States is 3–4 years longer than in Chinese women. American women are exposed to almost more than a decade of female hormones than Chinese women. Breast cancer incidence in Chinese women is one-fifth of that for American women. The China study consequently determined there was a very strong link between cancer and animal protein intake.

Dietary fiber and antioxidants have also been found linked to cancer occurrence. Because fiber and antioxidants are found mainly in plant foods, the average Chinese diet has three times more fiber and more antioxidants than the diet of many Americans. Results from the China study indicated that high fiber intake was associated with lower rates of colon and rectal cancers as well as lower blood cholesterol levels. Higher blood levels of the antioxidant vitamin C were also found to lower cancer rates. Low vitamin C levels are associated with breast, colon, esophageal, leukemia, liver, lung, nasopharynx, stomach, and rectal cancers. Other antioxidants, such as vitamin E and beta-carotene found in many plant foods, show a protective effect against damaging free radicals that increase the risk for cancers.

Obesity is another common problem in westernized societies. Americans in particular have tried a number of different weight loss diets, such as Atkins, South Beach, Paleo, and Weight Watcher's, in an effort to support weight loss toward a healthy weight. These diets all have a low carbohydrate approach, indicating that higher protein and fat diets are healthier than higher carbohydrate diets. However, the Chinese diet was found to be low in protein (90 percent of which is plant based) and fat and higher in carbohydrates and calories than westernized diets. Yet the Chinese have lower body weights and obesity rates when compared to westerners.

Overall, the China study concluded that while absolute proof in science is nearly impossible, the preponderance of evidence from this study and others clearly shows that a plant-based diet significantly reduces cancer, heart disease, and obesity. The final conclusions of the China Project were published in *The China Study: Revised and Expanded Edition* by T. Colin Campbell and Thomas M. Campbell in 2016. The T. Colin Campbell Center for Nutrition Studies also has a website (www.nutritionstudies .org) that educates the public about the benefits of plant-based diets and assists individuals with changing their diet habits.

13. Can plant-based diets benefit those with cardiovascular disease?

During the 1940s, cardiovascular disease was first identified as the major cause of mortality for many Americans. Cardiovascular diseases (CVD) are a group of disorders that affect the heart (coronary heart disease, rheumatic, congenital), brain (cerebrovascular disease or stroke), and blood circulation (peripheral artery disease, deep vein thrombosis). CVDs are the leading cause of death in most developed and affluent countries worldwide. As of 2017, the World Health Organization (WHO) estimates 17.9 million people die each year from cardiovascular disease, accounting for 31 percent of all deaths globally. WHO also estimates that 85 percent of deaths from CVDs are caused by either a heart attack or stroke.

After President Franklin Delano Roosevelt died from heart failure in 1945 due to undiagnosed heart disease, President Harry Truman signed into law the National Heart Act (1948), which declared, "Congress herby finds and declares the Nation's health is seriously threatened by diseases of the heart and circulation." This led to the creation of one of the most comprehensive and ongoing studies of CVDs, the Framingham Heart Study (FHS), and the creation of the National Heart, Lung, and Blood Institute.

Dr. Paul Dudley White, of Massachusetts General Hospital, and Dr. David Rutstein, of Harvard Medical School, pioneered the FHS. The FHS investigated residents who lived in Framingham, Massachusetts, because its population was representative of most Americans in the 1940s. It was also in close proximity to Harvard Medical School cardiologists. Since 1948, three generations of study participants have been tracked every two years and continue to be analyzed to the present day. In 1957, initial study results identified blood pressure, body weight, and cholesterol levels as primary risk factors for CVDs. As lab technology advanced over the years and study participants and their families were followed over time, specific blood lipid levels were further identified as risk factors for CVDs, and an association was also made between heart disease and diabetes.

The FHS confirmed that being overweight or obese, smoking tobacco, having high blood pressure, physical inactivity, elevated cholesterol levels, high uric acid levels, high blood sugar, and a diet high in saturated fats and sugars that was also low in the recommended amounts of vegetables, fruits, low-fat dairy, and whole grains, increased the risk for CVD incidence. Elevated levels of blood homocysteine (which indicates B vitamin deficiencies) were later identified as also increasing CVD risk. Genetic links were determined to be a minimal risk factor because those with similar genetic backgrounds, but different dietary habits, had different rates of CVDs. For example, Japanese men who lived in the United States had much higher blood cholesterol levels than Japanese men living in Japan. While having similar genetic backgrounds, diet differences appeared to play a more significant role in the cholesterol differences between the groups.

Before the FHS, it was generally accepted that CVDs were an inevitable fact of aging and little could be done about changing it. What became clear from the FHS and many subsequent studies is that saturated fats and cholesterol have a significant impact on heart health for many people worldwide. An aggressive campaign in the United States by public health officials educating Americans about tobacco use, low-fat and low-cholesterol diets, and exercise along with aggressive medical interventions, such as bypass surgeries and use of cardiac medications, contributed to an estimated 72 percent decline in coronary heart disease and 78 percent decline in strokes between 1950 and 2008. By 1984, The Framingham Nutrition Study (an offshoot of the FHS) results shaped many of the public health cardiovascular and nutrition guidelines recommended in the United States today.

However, the relationship between animal-based protein and plant-based protein was largely overlooked in these public health efforts. In 1985, Dr. Caldwell Esselstyn, a cardiologist at the world-renowned Wellness Institute at the Cleveland Clinic, treated his patients with a very low-fat plant-based protein diet. Only a minimal amount of cholesterol lowering medications was prescribed to his patients. All animal-based foods were eliminated. The goal of Dr. Esselstyn's program was to determine if a plant-based diet plan could prevent or reverse advanced coronary artery disease. The diet plan included flax seeds, whole grains, legumes, lentils, vegetables, and fruit. Multivitamins and vitamin B_{12} supplements were also recommended to prevent any unintentional nutritional deficiencies. All added oils, processed foods, avocado, nuts, excess salt, sugar, refined carbohydrates, caffeine, and animal-based foods were eliminated. Exercise was encouraged but not a requirement. One hundred ninety-eight patients, mostly men, were counseled about their diet during a five-hour program, and 89 percent faithfully followed this diet plan during the study period. Results were dramatic. Ninety-three percent of patients experienced improvement or resolution of their symptoms. One patient, who had restricted blood flood in his arteries, improved after three weeks to a normal blood flow and reduction in artery restriction. Twenty-two percent experienced a reversal in their disease process. Average weight loss for the group was approximately 19 pounds. The study concluded that plant-based nutrition could prevent, halt, and reverse coronary artery disease along with lifestyle modifications and cardiac medications.

Dr. Dean Ornish, who studied at Harvard Medical School, is also well known for his research in heart disease and diet. Dr. Ornish's Lifestyle Heart Trial examined 28 patients with heart disease. One group of patients was put on a low-fat plant-based diet along with stress management training, prohibition of tobacco use, and an exercise program of at least three days per week for one year. Patients attended biweekly meetings for support. The diet included fruit, vegetables, and grains. No animal foods were allowed except for egg whites and one cup of nonfat milk or yogurt daily. No medications or cardiac surgeries were prescribed for patients during this time period. The second group of 20 patients followed a standard cardiac treatment plan. The standard cardiac diet encourages a diet of moderation, which is low in cholesterol and allows no more than 7 percent of total calories from saturated fats and no more than 30 percent of total calories from fat. Recommendations advise maintaining blood cholesterol levels below 200 ml/dl. Patients eating the plant-based diet reduced their cholesterol levels from an average of 227 mg/dl to 172 mg/dl. They also reduced their low-density lipoprotein (LDL) cholesterol levels, which causes a buildup of cholesterol in arteries and is considered "bad" cholesterol, from 152 mg/dl to 95 mg/dl. Symptom severity improved and blockages in their arteries improved by 4 percent. After one year, 82 percent of the patients showed regression in their heart disease. However, the second group following the traditional cardiac diet experienced worsening symptoms and cholesterol levels, with an increase of blockages by 8 percent in the most noncompliant patients.

Although the Lifestyle Heart Trial was a small study, the premise that plant-based diets reduce CVDs has been upheld in other studies. For example, Dr. Francesca L. Crowe and colleagues in 2013 studied 44,561 men and women living in England and Scotland for a period of almost 12 years. Thirty-four percent of participants followed a vegetarian diet at the start of the study. The vegetarian group was found to have lower BMIs, blood pressures, and nonhigh density lipoprotein cholesterol (HDL-C) levels than the nonvegetarian group. The study also found the vegetarian group had a 32 percent lower risk for ischemic heart disease.

The Lyon Diet Heart Study (de Lorgeril) followed heart patients who ate a plant-based Mediterranean diet over a four-year time period. This study found that the Mediterranean diet was cardio protective, although medications were also prescribed as part of a comprehensive treatment plan. Researcher R. B. Singh found that individuals who ate a low-fat plant-based diet were more likely to have lower overall mortality, lower rates of myocardial infarction, and lower lipid blood levels than those who followed only a low-fat diet.

However, one study that does not uphold the conclusion of many other studies about plant-based diets, but warrants further investigation, is the Prospective Urban Rural Epidemiology (PURE) study. The PURE study is one of the largest studies of individuals between the ages of 35 and 70 investigating the relationship between diet, cardiovascular disease, and mortality in 18 countries. Between January 2003 and March 2013, 135,335 individuals were enrolled in the study and followed for an average of seven years. Diet analysis (using food frequency questionnaires) was compared with cardiac events (fatal and nonfatal heart attacks, stroke, and heart failure). Associations were made between consumption of carbohydrates, total fat, and type of fat and CVD events. The PURE study found high carbohydrate intake was associated with an increased risk for overall mortality, but not CVD risk or mortality. Total fat and types of fat intakes were also associated with lower risk of overall mortality. Higher intakes of saturated fat were found to lower the risk for stroke, but total fat and unsaturated fat had no statistically significant impact on risk for heart attack or CVD mortality. Many integrative medical practitioners believe fats have been unfairly maligned and have more health benefits than previously recognized. Given the scope of this study, further investigation is warranted.

14. Can plant-based diets benefit those with diabetes?

The pancreas is an important bodily organ and critical for control of blood sugar levels. An elevated blood sugar level, also known as hyperglycemia, is a common symptom of diabetes and can seriously damage many body organs over time. WHO estimated in 2014 that 8.5 percent of adults 18 years and older had diabetes worldwide. They also attributed an estimated 1.6 million deaths due to diabetic complications, making it the seventh leading cause of death in 2016 globally. The number of people with diabetes has risen from 108 million in 1980 to 422 million in 2014.

There are two types of diabetes, type 1 and type 2. Type 1, sometimes called juvenile onset diabetes, usually develops in children and adolescents and is connected with autoimmunity diseases and genetics. This form accounts for 5–10 percent of all diabetes cases and is due to an inability of the pancreas to make enough insulin, which is a hormone used to regulate blood sugars. Type 2, also called adult onset diabetes, accounts for 90–95 percent of all diabetes cases and usually occurs in adults over the age of 40. A new classification of diabetes, unofficially known as type 3, was recently designated as having a connection to Alzheimer's and the gene variant APOE4. Mayo Clinic researchers discovered that the APOE4 gene affects the ability of human brain cells to use insulin. In a currently ongoing study with the NIH, researchers identified study participants who had an APOE4 gene variation to have a reduced ability to use insulin in their brain, causing the cells to die. Those with an APOE4 gene variant were 10–15 times more likely to develop Alzheimer's disease. WHO estimates 50 million people worldwide have dementia and Alzheimer's disease accounts for 60–70 percent of dementia cases. Dementia is considered to be the major cause of disability and dependency worldwide.

Diet has always been an important component of diabetes prevention and treatment. When carbohydrate foods are eaten, the body produces insulin to turn glucose from carbohydrates into a usable energy form. Because insulin production is absent or compromised in diabetics, carbo-hydrate foods have the most impact on blood glucose levels. The tradi-tional diabetic diet has long recommended the elimination of processed foods and simple sugars from the diet, weight loss when needed, and reducing the amount of total carbohydrate foods eaten daily. In general, the American Diabetes Association and health care professionals counsel individuals with type 1 or 2 diabetes to eat only 45 percent of their total daily calories from carbohydrate foods that are also high in fiber, such as vegetables, fruit, legumes, low-fat dairy, and whole grain sources. The total amount of daily fat eaten, especially saturated fats, is restricted to no more than 30 percent of total calories because of the strong connection diabetes has with heart disease.

However, as researchers increasingly focus on plant-based diets, a num-ber of large studies have investigated the impact plant-based diets have on the prevention and treatment of diabetes. Most of these studies indicate that those who follow a mainly plant-based diet have lower body weight and lower rates of diabetes when compared to meat eaters and semiveg-etarians. The Adventist Health Study-2 (AHS-2) is one research effort that studied a large number of individuals who ate a plant-based diet over a long period of time. The AHS-2 study followed over 73,000 men and women from the United States and Canada from 2002 to 2007. Seventh Day Adventists were chosen because they follow a lacto-ovo vegetarian or vegan diet that avoids all meat for religious reasons. This study found that vegans had the lowest risk for diabetes when compared to lacto-ovo veg-etarians, pescovegetarians, semivegetarians, and nonvegetarians. Type 2 diabetes risk was reduced by 4 percent in vegans when compared to non-vegetarians. The study concluded that while variations of vegetarian diets do help reduce diabetes risk when compared to animal-based diets, the vegan meal plan had the greatest impact on reducing diabetes risk.

One of the most striking studies investigating the connection between diet and diabetes involves the Pima Indians who live in Arizona. The Pima Indians of the Gila River Indian Community have been studied since 1965 because they have the highest reported incidence of type 2 diabetes and obesity of any population in the world. Although type 1 diabetes is rare in the Pima Indians, it has been discovered that there is a genetic component in some Pima families influencing type I diabe-tes susceptibility. However, diet and environment appear to play a larger role than genetics due to the fact that 38 percent of Pima Indians in the United States have type 2 diabetes while 7 percent of Mexican Pima Indians have type 2 diabetes. The lower rate of diabetes and obesity in

Mexican Pima Indians suggests that even when there is a genetic suscep-tibility to diabetes, diet and environment can significantly impact risk for becoming a diabetic.

High rates of obesity and diabetes among the U.S. Pima Indians are attributed to the westernized diet many American Pima Indians eat. The traditional diet of the Pima Indians is high in fiber and whole grain car-bohydrates while lower in fat than the modern Pima diet that has adapted to a westernized way of eating. Traditional Pima diets are estimated to be 70–80 percent of calories from whole grain carbohydrates, 12–18 percent from plant-based proteins (although animal proteins were not excluded), and 8–12 percent from fat. Dietary studies found when Pima study subjects returned to eating a traditional diet of beans, corns, grains, greens, mes-quite, tepary beans, and other low fiber plant foods, blood sugars returned to normal levels and weight loss occurred.

15. How can plant-based diets affect an individual's weight?

Being overweight or obese is closely associated with many chronic diseases and life expectancy of westernized societies. In 2008, WHO estimated 23 percent of women and 20 percent of men were obese (defined as having a body mass index or BMI of 30.0 or higher) in the European region. This number doubled between 1980 and 2008. They also estimated that over 50 percent of men and women were overweight (defined as having a BMI between 25 and 30). BMI is a tool used to measure body fat of adults based on their height and weight and assists health professionals to determine healthy weight status. In the United States, the 2013–14 NHANES study found more than 33 percent of adults were overweight and over 33 percent were obese. The NHANES also found 17 percent of children and adolescents, aged 2–19, were considered obese putting them at an increased risk to be overweight or obese as adults.

Many adults and children struggle to lose weight to normal levels. Sub-optimal eating habits and reduced activity levels are closely associated with weight gain. A number of diets and exercise programs have evolved over the years in the quest for an effective weight loss program. In 2014, the weight loss industry in the United States was a $64 billion market. Plant-based diets have become the latest solution for promoting weight loss. But do they really work? A variety of studies and reviews indicate that plant-based diets can be an effective strategy for weight reduction and the prevention of obesity because they are low in energy density and high in complex carbohydrates, fiber, and water.

Susan E. Berkow, PhD, CNS, and Neal Barnard, MD, researchers with the Physicians Committee for Responsible Medicine, identified 40 observational studies that analyzed weight and BMI differences between vegetarians and nonvegetarians. Twenty-nine studies found vegetarians weighed significantly less and had lower BMIs than nonvegetarians. Data results were adjusted for smoking and exercise habits that would also affect the results.

In 2016, researchers R. Y. Huang, C. C. Huang, F. B. Hu, and J. E. Chavarro analyzed 12 studies involving over 1,100 individuals divided into vegan, vegetarian, and nonvegetarian diet groups. Study results found that those who followed a vegan diet had the most weight loss of all three groups. Both the vegan and vegetarian groups lost more weight than the nonvegetarian group.

In 2006, S. E. Berkow and N. Barnard found vegan and vegetarian diets were highly effective weight loss diets, with a simultaneous decrease in risk for heart disease, high blood pressure, diabetes, and obesity. They also concluded that those who ate a vegan diet burned more calories after meals in comparison to nonvegans who burned fewer calories.

The Adventist Health Study-2, discussed in Question 12, also studied obesity levels in Seventh Day Adventist adults. Study results found vegetarian diets promoted weight loss and helped to prevent obesity.

The European Prospective Investigation into Cancer and Nutrition (EPIC) is another large cohort study that analyzed more than half a million participants worldwide in ten European countries over a 15-year time span. The EPIC study investigated the relationship between nutrition status, diet, lifestyle, and environment. While their primary focus was on the relationship between diet and cancer and other chronic disease, study results also found individuals who ate meat had higher BMIs than vegans, who had the lowest BMIs. BMIs of vegetarians ranged between the meat eaters and vegans.

Besides the concern of being overweight or obese, being too thin can also be detrimental for health. Being underweight is associated with malnourishment and premature death. Other lifestyle risk factors associated with being underweight also include drug and alcohol abuse, mental health issues, poverty, and tobacco use. Those who are underweight (defined as having a BMI of 18.5 or lower) have a 1.8 greater chance of premature death when compared to normal weight individuals. Those who are overweight have a 1.2 greater chance, and those are severely obese have a 1.3 greater chance of premature death when compared to normal weight individuals. According to the T. Colin Campbell Center for Nutrition Studies, 1.4 percent of U.S adults over the age of 20 were underweight in 2014.

For normal weight individuals switching to a plant-based diet, there is an increased risk for becoming underweight if the diet is not properly planned. As discussed in previous questions, most individuals have a tendency to eat an abundance of vegetables and carbohydrates but neglect to eat adequate protein and fat. Foods that are high in protein and fat have more calories as a rule than vegetables, fruits, and complex carbohydrates. Portion sizes of food are often decreased, which also reduces calories and contributes to weight loss. As reported in the March 2014 issue of the journal *Nutrients*, researchers comparing the nutritional quality of vegan, vegetarian, semivegetarian, pescovegetarian, and omnivorous diets found vegans had the most restricted total calorie and protein intake with the highest amount of sugar, carbohydrates, and fiber intake when compared to all other groups. However, they also found that all diet groups (except meat eaters) had the same number of underweight individuals, which ranged from 6 percent to 9 percent, when compared to 3 percent of omnivores.

16. Do plant-based diets increase life expectancy?

Life expectancy, or longevity, is defined as the average number of years an individual is expected to live. Life expectancy has steadily increased since the early 1900s and is impacted by a number of factors, such as gender, genetics, prenatal and childhood environment, marital and socioeconomic status, education, ethnicity, lifestyle, and diet. As of 2016, WHO estimated the average life expectancy of humans around the globe was 72 years of age. This is further broken down into age 74 for females and 69.8 years for males. The World Factbook, which is compiled by the U.S. Central Intelligence Agency (CIA), provides more detailed estimates of average life expectancy by country. A snapshot of life expectancy in developed countries versus developing countries is as follows: Monaco 89.4 years of age; Japan 85.3; Hong Kong 83; Switzerland 82.6; Israel 82.5; Australia 82.3; Italy 82.3; Sweden 82.1; France 81.9; Norway 81.9; Canada 81.9; Spain 81.8; Ireland 80.9; Germany 80.8; Greece 80.7; United States 80; United Arab Emirates 77.7; Argentina 77.3; Mexico 76.1; China 75.7; Saudi Arabia 75.5; Turkey 75; Brazil 74; Russia 71; India 68.8; Kenya 64; Haiti 64; Afghanistan 51.7; and Chad 50.6.

While there are many factors that affect longevity, nutrition and lifestyle habits appear to play the most important role in how long a person lives. The emergence of blue zones appears to support this theory. Dan Buettner, a National Geographic Fellow, defined and reported about blue zones in 2004 after discovering the work of Michel Poulain, who was studying centenarians. Centenarians are individuals who live to be 100 or more years of age. Michel Poulain and his colleagues found the number of centenarians in Sardinia, Italy, was significantly higher than those in other European countries—16.6 per 100,000 inhabitants in Sardinia versus 10 per 100,000 in other European countries. Men also lived longer in Sardinia than they did elsewhere, with the female/male ratio being 2:1 in Sardinia versus 5:1 in other countries. Poulain and his colleagues wanted to confirm that factors in Sardinia influenced the increased life span of men and that geographical distribution of centenarians is nonrandom and specific to Sardinia. They were able to confirm, after analyzing their data, that the Sardinian population had a significantly increased likelihood of living longer, especially men, and that nutrition and lifestyle along with climate and cultural features of this area were the key factors behind increased longevity.

Blue zone characteristics are defined by researchers (the term "blue zone" originating from the fact that a blue marker was used to distinguish it on a map) as an area that has decreased accessibility for many decades, usually because they are located in a mountainous region. This decreased geographic accessibility reduced the impact of immigration, which increases intermarriage. Thus, the majority of Sardinians were descended from a common ancestor, reducing genetic variability, and their "healthy" nutrition and lifestyle habits were preserved. Sardinians remained genetically isolated over time and their cultural and lifestyle habits have been unchanged for a number of centuries, making research findings significant.

Dan Buettner reported about Poulain's work and identified the five geographic locations where people live the longest and are the healthiest in the world as blue zones. These blue zones are Okinawa, Japan; Sardinia, Italy; Nicoya, Costa Rica; Ikaria, Greece; and Loma Linda, California. All blue zones share nine specific characteristics. Individuals living in these zones move all day long—either gardening or performing yard or housework. They do not have programmed exercise routines, such as going to gyms or run marathons. They also have a sense of purpose in their life. They reduce stress in their daily life by meditating or taking naps or just relaxing. They follow the 80 percent rule, which is the practice of eating only until they are 80 percent full at meals and eating their smallest meal in the late afternoon or early evening with no snacking in the evening. Plant-based diets are the foundation of their nutritional intake, and vegetables and legumes are the main staple of their diet. Only three to four ounces of meat are eaten five times per month. Wine is a regular drink in moderation, with no more than one to two glasses per day. All belong to faith-based communities, which are shown to add 4–14 years onto life expectancy. Family also comes first, and their societies are plentiful in social networks that support healthy behaviors.

In addition to Poulain's work, research also finds that diet is instrumental in increasing life expectancy. In 2013, the Global Burden of Disease Study investigated 79 different factors that determined death and disability of individuals in 188 countries from 1990 to 2013. This study concluded that poor diet was associated with over 11 million deaths and was the major cause of disability. A similar study in the United States in 2014 determined that poor diet was associated with 26 percent of all deaths.

So, what type of diet has been found to contribute to a longer life span? A review of nutrition studies (reported in *The Journal of Nutrition* in 2014) found those who ate a modified Mediterranean Diet, DASH diet (Dietary Approaches to Stop Hypertension), or closely followed the recommendations of the Dietary Guidelines for Americans—(all plant-based diets low in sodium, saturated fat, sugar, and red or processed meats) experienced lower rates of mortality. Although none of these diets eliminate dairy or other animal foods, all recommend vegetables, fruits, legumes, and healthy fats as the foundation of the daily diet.

In 2019, study results focusing on the long-term effects of high dietary protein intakes for all-cause mortalities were published in the *JAMA Internal Medicine* journal. This study followed 70,696 Japanese participants, aged 45–74 years, who had no history of cancer or CVDs over a 20-year period. Researchers found that participants who ate mostly plant proteins in their diet were 13 percent less likely to die during the study and 16 percent less likely to die of CVDS. Individuals who replaced 3 percent of the red meat they ate with plant protein were 34 percent less likely to die from all-cause mortality, 39 percent less likely to die from cancer, and 42 percent less likely to die from CVDs. Those who replaced 4 percent of their red meat intake with plant protein were 46 percent less likely to die of all-cause mortality and 50 percent less likely to die from cancer. However, it should be noted that study participants diet habits were only assessed at the beginning of the study and not reevaluated over the 20-year study period, increasing the chance of unaccounted for diet habits.

17. Why do some people become unhealthy when following a plant-based diet?

Many people assume that vegan and vegetarian diets are healthy and perfectly balanced nutritionally. However, that is the furthest thing from the truth. Many processed, plant-based foods tend to be high in sodium, saturated fat, sugars, and calories. A good example of this is the popularity of plant-based meat alternatives. There are many different brand name meat alternative products. Until 2019, the majority of these meat alternatives were made from limited ingredients and tasted like a plant-based meat. As people have become more health and environmentally conscious, the demand for meat alternatives that taste and look like meat has increased. A number of new plant-based processed meats have recently become available and people assume they are a healthier alternative to meat. But that isn't always the case nutritionally.

Original plant-based burgers, such as NEAT veggie burgers, contain pecans, garbanzo beans, gluten free whole grain oats, organic gluten free whole grain cornmeal, chia seeds, spices, onion, garlic, and sea salt. Nutritionally NEAT veggie burgers are 10 percent sodium, 8 percent saturated fat, and 140 calories per burger. The updated version of plant-based burgers that reportedly taste just like meat and even "bleed" like red meat contains far more ingredients and is not as healthy as assumed. The ingredients for Beyond Meat burgers are water, pea protein isolate, expeller-pressed canola oil, refined coconut oil, rice protein, natural flavors, cocoa butter, mung bean protein, methylcellulose, potato starch, apple extract, salt, potassium chloride, vinegar, lemon juice concentrate, sunflower lecithin, pomegranate fruit powder, and beet juice extract. Nutritionally Beyond Meat burgers provide 15 percent sodium, 25 percent saturated fat, and 260 calories per burger.

Plant-based diets also include foods, such as legumes, nuts, and seeds, which are calorically dense. Calorically dense foods provide more calories and nutritional value in a smaller portion size when compared to most other foods. Many people assume that because all plant-based foods are "healthy," they can eat as much as desired and tend to overconsume recommended portion sizes. This in turn leads to overconsuming calories that can cause weight gain. Choosing french fries, cookies, and processed carbohydrate foods, such as potato or vegetable chips, can be high in saturated fats, sugars, and calories that negatively impact both health and weight.

Nutritional deficiencies can also occur when a food group is eliminated or reduced in the diet. Vegans are especially vulnerable since they eliminate all animal foods, which can lead to nutritional deficiencies. For example, vegans and vegetarians tend to be deficient in vitamins B_{12} and D, calcium, omega-3 fatty-acids, zinc, and iron—all nutrients found in meat and not available in large enough amounts in plant foods to prevent deficiencies. Long-term deficiencies of these nutrients can result in illness or chronic disease over time. Weight loss and hair loss are two common problems for vegans as the result of poor diet planning and resulting nutrition deficiencies. Researchers at the Harvard T.H. Chan School of Public Health found that plant-based diets low in animal foods were linked with a 20 percent lower risk for diabetes. However, those who ate less healthy plant foods actually increased their risk for diabetes by 16 percent. Careful meal planning is essential when following a plant-based diet and will be discussed in depth in Questions 18 and 19.

Even with careful nutritionally planning, some people do not respond well physically when they eat a vegetarian or vegan meal plan and need to include some animal-based foods in their diet for good health. No one really understands yet the reason for this, but it would appear that genetics may play a key role. In Question 10, Dr. Peter J. D'Adamo's blood type diet was discussed. While the diet is not taken seriously, Dr. D'Adamo posits that specific blood types based on genetics require animal-based foods for good health. An insufficient number of studies have been done to date to either confirm or discredit his theories. However, more research into this area may provide an answer to this puzzling reaction. Health and bacterial makeup of the gastrointestinal microbiome, ability to digest plants, or undiagnosed individual food allergies/sensitivities may also play a role in how well a person tolerates a plant-based diet. Medical conditions and individual negative or allergic reactions to plant-based foods are further discussed in Questions 22 and 23.

Nutritional Management of Plant-Based Diets

18. What are the most important nutrition guidelines to follow to maintain good health when eating vegan or vegetarian?

No matter what diet a person eats, it is always important to become educated about nutrition and how to eat a nutritionally balanced diet that maintains good health. Food, in the proper amounts and balance, provides energy and essential nutrients for survival as well as for the development, growth, and future health of an unborn child. Plant-based diets eliminate most animal foods. Eliminating any food group from the daily diet can be problematic because every food group has nutritional benefits. However, these potential nutrient deficiencies can be avoided with careful meal planning and supplementation when necessary. To understand potential nutrition and health risks, it is important to review basic nutrition concepts.

While there are numerous elements in foods that are important, the most important food nutrients are classified as macronutrients and micronutrients. Macronutrients provide energy that helps the body to function and are categorized as carbohydrates, proteins, and fats. Carbohydrates fuel the body by providing energy. There are two types of carbohydrates: simple and complex. Simple carbohydrates require little digestion and supply a fast-usable energy source. Complex carbohydrates require more time and effort to break down into a form the body can use for energy. Nutritionally, complex carbohydrates are superior to simple carbohydrates as they supply fiber and are a better source of vitamins, minerals, and phytochemicals. Protein supplies energy, but its primary role is to provide amino acids. Amino acids are necessary for growth, repair, and maintenance of body tissues and muscles. Protein also supports the immune system's ability to fight infections, supports decreased inflammation, and is critical for fetal growth and development. Fats, also called lipids, are important sources of fatty acids and supply energy for the body to use. Fatty acids are necessary to absorb fat-soluble vitamins and are used in many biological processes. Research shows that "healthy" fats are critical for the formation of the brain, eyes, and nervous system during fetal growth. Fatty acids are also essential for growth and good health throughout the life cycle.

Micronutrients are commonly known as vitamins and minerals and act as cofactors in biological processes essential for normal growth, metabolism, and health. Vitamins and minerals are the "spark plugs" that ignite the "fuel" in food, controlling the critical functions used by the body to make the body "run" smoothly and efficiently. Suboptimal intake of essential micronutrients will result in poor health and chronic illnesses. Micronutrients are just as important as macronutrients for good health. The essential vitamins and minerals every human require to stay health are summarized in Table 1.

The Institute of Medicine (IOM) in the United States established minimum and maximum recommended daily dietary amounts for each vitamin and mineral based on available evidence and scientific judgment. Known as the Dietary Reference Intakes (DRIs), they are formulated for healthy individuals. Individuals with chronic or compromised health conditions may require increased recommended amounts.

There are six main food groups important for maintaining good health: dairy, fats, fruits, grains, protein, and vegetables. Each food group has important health benefits, and each group is interconnected nutritionally, often providing enhanced nutrition benefits when eaten together. Eliminating any food group can have a significant impact on health. The most common nutrient deficiencies and symptoms among vegans and vegetarians are summarized in Table 2.

Risk for a nutritional deficiency is determined by the type of plant-based diet selected and overall diet habits. Vegans have the highest risk for nutrient deficiencies. Those who include some animal foods in their diets have a lower risk, but they still need to be aware of ensuring adequate nutrient intake.

Table 1   Essential vitamins and minerals

Vitamins	
Fat-soluble	Water-soluble
A	Vitamin B_1 (thiamine)
D	Vitamin B_2 (riboflavin)
E	Vitamin B_3 (niacin)
K	Vitamin B_5 (pantothenic acid)
	Vitamin B_6 (pyridoxine)
	Vitamin B_9 (folate or folic acid)
	Vitamin B_{12} (cobalamins)
	Biotin (also a B vitamin)
	Vitamin C
	Choline
Minerals	
Macrominerals	Trace minerals
Calcium	Copper
Chloride	Fluoride
Magnesium	Iodine
Phosphorus	Iron
Potassium	Manganese
Sodium	Nickel
	Selenium
	Zinc

The most effective solution to ensure a well-balanced diet nutritionally is meeting with an experienced health professional specializing in nutrition, such as a registered dietitian. Registered dietitians (RDs) or registered nutritionists (RDNs) are health care professionals who receive a bachelor's degree in food and nutrition, complete an accredited and supervised nutrition practice program, and pass a national certification exam to become RDs. To maintain their certification as nutrition specialists, they are required to complete continuing education programs throughout their career. Meeting with an RD or RDN includes a review of diet habits and eating patterns, analysis of nutrient intake, identification of potential deficiencies, review of dietary supplement needs, and the formation

Table 2   Common nutrient deficiencies among vegans and vegetarians

Nutrient	Food group	Function	Vegetarian/ Vegan alternative food options	Some potential risks from deficiency
Vitamin D	Dairy	Promotes calcium absorption in the GI tract and maintains bone mineralization	Fortified milk drinks and juices, margarine, sun exposure (15 minutes daily, without sunscreen)	Bone or tooth fractures, osteoporosis, severe asthma in children
Riboflavin	Dairy, eggs	Metabolizes carbohydrates, fats, and protein to produce energy	Grains, leafy green vegetables	Heart and orofacial cleft birth defects, sore throat, cheilosis
Vitamin B_{12}	Dairy, eggs, meat	Makes DNA and nerve and blood cells	Fortified breakfast cereals, nutritional yeasts, dietary supplements	Blindness, fatigue, gastritis, gastrointestinal disorders, pernicious anemia, immune system disorders, muscle weakness
Calcium	Dairy	Maintains bone and heart health, necessary for muscle contractions	Beans, calcium-fortified drinks or foods, leafy green vegetables, dairy foods	Bone and tooth fractures, osteopenia, weakness and fatigue, delayed growth in children, blood pressure regulation disorders

Table 2 Continued

Nutrient	Food group	Function	Vegetarian/ Vegan alternative food options	Some potential risks from deficiency
Iron	Meat	Essential component of red blood cells; required for physical growth, hormone synthesis, and neurological development	Beans, dried fruits, iron-fortified grains, dietary supplements	Anemia, fatigue, fetal cretinism and mental retardation
Omega-3s	Fish, krill, seafood	Form cell membranes; fetal brain formation; brain, eye, sperm health	Algae, flax seeds, canola and soybean oils, dietary supplements	Increased risk for cancer, CVDs, age-related macular degeneration, scaly red itchy rash
Zinc	Meat, dairy, fish, shellfish	Supports the immune system, makes DNA, fetal growth and development, proper sense of taste and smell	Fortified cereals, legumes, whole grains	Decreased stress tolerance, poor wound healing, decreased immunity

SOURCE: National Institutes of Health, Office of Dietary Supplements.

of a specific and individualized diet plan to meet daily nutrition needs that can help a person transition to a plant-based diet. There are also many web-based resources that can assist an individual to maintain adequate nutritional health. The International Vegan Association publishes a Vegan Starter Kit and the Physicians Committee for Responsible Medicine publishes a Vegetarian Starter Kit. Both kits explain the rationale for their respective diets and provide helpful guidelines to transition to the diet. Both kits are available on their websites. Other reputable resources are included in Question 31.

19. What nutritional deficiencies can develop while following a plant-based diet?

As discussed in Question 18, when any food group is eliminated from the diet, nutritional deficiencies can occur. Vegans are at the highest risk for nutrition deficiencies because all animal foods are eliminated from the diet. Vegetarians are at less risk since some animal foods are still included in their diet. However, unless both groups carefully plan their meals, they can become deficient in protein, minerals, and vitamins, having the potential for negative health consequences. The most common nutrition deficiencies vegans and vegetarians are at risk for include protein, calcium, iron, omega-3s, vitamins B_{12} and D and riboflavin, and zinc.

Amino acids make up the macronutrient protein. Proteins are essential for the manufacture of enzymes and hormones and the structure, function, and regulation of body cells, tissues, and organs. Each protein has a unique function that is also responsible for growth and maintenance of muscles and tissues, transport of nutrients, and fluid balance, among other things. Those who eat plant-based diets are at risk for protein deficiencies. A high-quality source of protein is considered a food that contains all essential amino acids. Amino acids are a group of organic molecules that combine to form proteins. Amino acids are considered the building blocks of life, and they are broken down into essential and nonessential categories. The body cannot make essential amino acids. As a result, they must be included in the daily diet. Essential amino acids are histidine, isoleucine, leucine, lysine, methionine, phenylalanine, threonine, tryptophan, and valine. However, the body can make its own nonessential amino acid supply. Therefore, daily nonessential amino acid food sources are not necessary. Nonessential amino acids are alanine, arginine, asparagine, aspartic acid, cysteine, glutamic acid, glutamine, glycine, proline, serine, and tyrosine. Foods that contain all essential amino acids in adequate amounts are beef, cheeses, chicken, eggs, fish, milk, turkey, and yogurt and classified as complete proteins. Plant-based foods that have a high-quality amino acid profile include buckwheat, Ezekiel bread, quinoa, soy and tofu. Beans, also known as legumes, are a good source of protein but must be combined with rice to provide all essential amino acids. This is because most beans are low in methionine and high in lysine. Rice is low in lysine and high in methionine. Therefore, eating them together provides a complete protein that is found in animal foods. Peanut butter is another example. Peanuts are a legume, so pairing them with whole wheat, such as in a sandwich, completes the protein profile making it a good protein food source. Symptoms of a protein deficiency include edema; mood changes; fingernail, hair, and skin disorders; fatigue and weakness; hunger; slow healing wounds; and frequent illnesses with a delayed recovery time.

Calcium is another important nutrient that must be included in the daily diet. Calcium is a macro mineral, meaning it is required in a larger amount daily in comparison to trace minerals, which are needed in smaller amounts for optimal health. Calcium is needed to maintain strong bones and teeth. It is also needed to assist blood vessels and muscles to contract and expand, to secrete hormones and enzymes, and to send messages throughout the nervous system. Calcium is found in dairy foods, such as cheese, fish with soft edible bones such as salmon and sardines, milk, and yogurt. Since most vegetarians include dairy foods in their diet, vegans are most at risk for calcium deficiencies. Plant-based sources of calcium include green, leafy vegetables, and calcium enriched cereals, fruit juices, rice and soy drinks, and tofu. Symptoms of a calcium deficiency include frequent bone fractures and osteoporosis.

Iron is a very important trace mineral. It is an essential component of hundreds of proteins and enzymes that support critical biological functions such as the transport of oxygen throughout the body, DNA synthesis, and energy production. It is also critical in the proper development of the fetus. There are two types of iron: heme and nonheme. Heme iron is found in fish, liver, red meat, and poultry. Nonheme iron is also found in meat, but it is mostly found in plant foods and dairy foods. Heme iron is well absorbed by the body, while nonheme iron is not as well absorbed and affected by other dietary foods that may be eaten at the same time. For example, vitamin C foods increase the absorption of nonheme iron, while phytic acid, found in legumes, whole grains, nuts, and seed, decreases nonheme iron absorption. Soy protein also decreases nonheme iron absorption. Symptoms of an iron deficiency include fatigue, rapid heart rate or palpitations, and shortness of breath. Severe iron deficiencies can cause difficulty swallowing, mouth sores, pica, and taste bud atrophy. Iron deficiencies during pregnancy can result in birth defects and will be further discussed in Question 20.

Omega-3s are essential fatty acids critical for fetal brain, eye, and central nervous system development. They are considered essential since the body cannot make them and is dependent on food sources for them. Adults also need them to maintain the integrity of cell membranes, for proper function of the cardiovascular and nervous systems, for adequate vision, and as an energy source. There are three forms of omega-3s: docosahexaenoic acid (DHA), eicosapentaenoic acid (EPA), and alpha-linolenic acid (ALA). The best food sources for omega-3s include fish and shellfish because they have high amounts of DHA and EPA. Plant sources of omega-3s, which have the ALA form of omega-3s, include canola oil, flaxseeds, chia seeds, black walnuts, and soybeans. However, it needs to be noted that ALA from plant foods are not converted well into DHA. This means higher amounts of ALA must be eaten to receive the health benefits of omega-3s. Symptoms of omega-3 deficiencies include dermatitis, learning and memory impairments, neuropathy and visual problems.

Vitamin B_{12} is an essential vitamin that keeps nerve and blood cells healthy and makes DNA. It is found in beef liver, clams, dairy foods, eggs, fish, red meat, and poultry. Plant food sources include fortified breakfast cereals and other fortified foods, and nutritional yeast. Symptoms of a vitamin B_{12} deficiency include megaloblastic anemia, loss of appetite, confusion and memory impairment, constipation, depression, fatigue, nerve damage, tingling in hands and feet, and weight loss.

Vitamin D is another important vitamin that supports strong bones and teeth by helping the body absorb calcium. It is also used by the nervous system to carry messages throughout the body and used by the immune system to fight off infection. The fetus requires it for formation of bones and teeth. The skin through sun exposure manufactures vitamin D. But depending on where one lives (higher latitudes can decrease the amount of vitamin D a person makes), food sources or dietary supplements are needed to maintain an adequate level of vitamin D. Food sources of vitamin D include dairy foods, fatty fish (salmon, tuna, mackerel), beef liver, cheese, and egg yolks. Plant food sources of vitamin D include mushrooms and vitamin D fortified foods. Vitamin D deficiencies increase the risk for osteoporosis and rickets, and they may also increase the risk for fetal growth retardation and low bone mineral density as well also some cancers.

Riboflavin, also known as vitamin B_2, is essential as a coenzyme in energy production, cell functions, cell growth and development, and the metabolism of fats and pharmaceutical drugs and steroids. Food sources of riboflavin are eggs, organ meats (kidney and liver), lean meat, and milk. Plant food sources include green vegetables and fortified cereals and breads. Symptoms of riboflavin deficiencies include skin diseases, edema of the mouth and throat, cheilosis or angular stomatitis, hair loss, reproductive problems, sore throat, degeneration of the liver and nervous system, and thyroid disorders. Long-term riboflavin deficiencies can cause anemia and cataracts.

Zinc is a trace mineral that has numerous functions. It is primarily found to assist the immune system in fighting infections and viruses as well as helps to make proteins and DNA. In the fetus, zinc is important for growth and development, immune and nervous system function, taste and smell, and protein formation. Food sources of zinc include beef, crab, dairy foods, lobster, poultry, and oysters. Plant food sources of zinc include beans, nuts, whole grains, and fortified breakfast cereals. Deficiencies of zinc include frequent illnesses, diarrhea, and age-related macular degeneration. In children, a deficiency can cause impaired behavior development and decreased stress tolerance.

20. Can pregnant women have a healthy baby while following a vegetarian or vegan diet?

The maternal diet has a prolonged and lasting impact on an unborn child. Questions 17, 18, and 19 explored the most common nutrient deficiencies that can occur when a plant-based diet is not properly planned. Because of the rapid growth and complexity of fetal development, any nutrient deficiency during pregnancy can negatively impact growth while also increasing the risk for birth complications and birth defects. All nutrients are important for fetal development, but there are certain nutrients that are specifically increased during pregnancy. According to the American College of Obstetricians and Gynecologists, the most critical nutrient needs during pregnancy are calcium, folate, iodine, iron, omega-3s, and vitamins A, B_6, B_{12}, C, and D. Deficiencies of any of these nutrients can significantly impact fetal development and long-term health. In addition to nutrients, total daily calorie intake may impact fetal health and development as well.

Fetal development is rapid. The embryonic stage, which begins at two weeks after fertilization, is a critical stage of development. The spinal column forms during the first four weeks of pregnancy. Folate (folic acid) deficiency during this time increases the risk for neural tube defects, such as spina bifida. Folate deficiency can also increase the risk for anencephaly, preeclampsia, premature delivery, low birth weight, small gestational age, and stillbirths. Plant-based sources of folate include asparagus, beets, broccoli, brussels sprouts, citrus fruit, eggs, leafy green vegetables, and legumes. Folate also has a symbiotic relationship with vitamin B_{12}. Maternal B_{12} stores are below acceptable levels in about 20 percent of normal pregnancies. However, because it is thought that this is a normal physiological process of pregnancy, rather than a deficiency, vitamin

B_{12} is usually not a vitamin aggressively supplemented during pregnancy. It has been found, though, that supplementing with folate or eating folate-fortified foods (normally prescribed for women of child bearing age who are considering becoming pregnant) can increase the risk for a vitamin B_{12} deficiency. Because of this risk, vitamin B_{12} is usually included in prenatal vitamins along with folate. Plant-based sources of vitamin B_{12} are outlined in Question 19.

Omega-3 fatty acids (DHA and EPA) are critical for proper brain, nervous system, and eye formation. The fetal and infant brain develops very rapidly during the last trimester of pregnancy and the first two years of life. But even at conception and through the first and second trimesters of pregnancy, the fetal brain is developing numerous new cells, synapses, and neurons. DHA is necessary for the growth of neurons and fetal needs for DHA actually doubles during intense brain growth periods. EPA is equally important because it assists DHA to cross the placental barrier where it is bound and taken up for use by fetal cells for brain formation. Plant-based sources of omega-3s are discussed in Question 19.

Both mother and baby need calcium for strong bones and teeth. Adequate calcium intake by the mother increases fetal bone mineral density, preserves the bone health of the mother, and decreases the risk for low birth weight babies and premature birth. Pregnant teenage moms are especially at risk for bone loss because they themselves are still growing and have increased calcium needs. Vitamin D supports the building of fetal and infant bones and teeth and maintains bone health of the mother by promoting calcium absorption. Vitamin D deficiencies may also increase the risk for fetal growth retardation and low bone mineral density. Both calcium and vitamin D plant-based foods are outlined in Question 19.

Deficiencies of iodine and iron can significantly impact IQ and increase risk for cretinism and mental retardation. Iodine deficiency during pregnancy is one of the most preventable causes of fetal brain damage around the world. Iodine requirements for women can increase more than 50 percent during pregnancy, so adequate iodine stores prior to pregnancy are important. Iodine deficiencies have been linked to cretinism in babies, which severely stunts physical and mental growth of the baby. Iodine deficiency is also one of the leading causes for fetal hypothyroidism, which can cause mental retardation. Mothers can develop thyroid disease if their iodine levels are low, which increases risk for premature birth, preeclampsia (severe high blood pressure), and low birth weight babies. Plant-based food sources of iodine include whole grains, green beans, kale, organic potatoes with skin, and strawberries.

Iron is a required mineral for many biochemical pathways to operate properly. It is an essential component for oxygen transport and the regulation of fetal cell growth and development into specialized cells. A deficiency in iron limits oxygen delivery to cells for the mother, resulting in anemia, fatigue, and decreased immunity. The growing baby also requires iron to grow and develop, especially during the second and third trimesters. Iron deficiency can impair fetal brain development and increase the risk for premature birth, low birth weight, and postpartum depression. Iron deficiencies are also associated with memory impairment and attention disorders in infants and young children. However, many women begin their pregnancy iron deficient. Caution must be used with iron supplements, however, because some people may have a genetic disorder known as hemochromatosis. Individuals with hemochromatosis store excess amounts of iron in their body tissues, which cause liver damage, diabetes, and a bronze discoloration of the skin and, if left untreated, can be fatal. Blood levels of iron should always be checked before supplements with iron are taken. Plant-based sources of iron are discussed in Question 19.

Vitamin A is important for growth and development of the fetus because of its involvement in growth, vision, protein synthesis, and cell differentiation. There are two forms of vitamin A in foods: preformed vitamin A (called retinols found in animal-sourced foods, i.e. dairy, fish, and meat) and pro-vitamin A (carotenoids, also called carotene, found in fruits and vegetables). The most important pro-vitamin A is beta-carotene. Beta-carotene and other carotenoids can be converted by the body into the active form of vitamin A used for biochemical reactions in the body. But carotenoids are only converted into vitamin A if the body needs it. Thus, carotenoids are a safer form of vitamin A to take and beta-carotene is the preferred form for use in dietary supplements to decrease a risk of vitamin A toxicity. Although vitamin A deficiency has been linked to increased risk for birth defects, vitamin A deficiency is rare in the United States.

Vitamin C is an important antioxidant for collagen and connective tissue formation, strong immunity, and wound healing. Low-income mothers are more likely to have vitamin C deficiencies, which can increase risk for premature births, urinary tract infections, or impaired healing. Vitamin C also helps to increase absorption of iron from foods and supplements. Vitamin C needs are increased even more for women who smoke because tobacco depletes body stores of vitamin C. Plant-based food sources of vitamin C include bell peppers, broccoli, brussels sprouts, kiwi, oranges, spinach, strawberries.

Vitamin B_6 plays a key role in cognitive development and is involved as a cofactor in many biochemical reactions. Deficiencies can increase inflammation in the body and increase risk for behavior abnormalities, low birth weight, and low APGAR scores in infants and young children. Women who have taken birth control pills or who smoke tobacco are at increased risk for vitamin B_6 deficiencies during pregnancy. Plant-based sources of vitamin B_6 include acorn squash, avocado, banana, fortified vegan cereals, quinoa, pistachio nuts, sunflower seeds, whole grain pasta, and wheat germ.

As can be seen, while all nutrients are important for the human body to form correctly and adequate brain and nerve development to occur, some nutrients are even more critical during certain phases of fetal development than others. WebMD has a very informative slideshow of the stages of fetal development.

Beside nutrient needs, calorie needs are also increased during pregnancy. This can become a concern because some mothers may not eat enough calories due to a preference for low-calorie plant-based foods. In general women require an extra 300 calories daily to support both mother and baby. With careful planning calorie needs and nutrient needs are easily met.

21. Is it safe for children to follow a vegetarian or vegan diet?

Like women, children have unique nutritional needs. Childhood is a period of rapid growth and development, so the right balance of nutrients in a child's daily diet is critically important for development and health well into adulthood. Proper nutritional planning supports the healthy growth of a child well into their adulthood.

Children double their weight within the first four to five months after birth. Healthy infants need about three times more calories per kilogram of body weight than adults to support growth. Growth spurts also occur during preschool ages and puberty. Therefore, calorie intake is very important during these growth periods, especially for premature infants who have even higher caloric needs. General guidelines estimate that children require between 1,000 and 1,400 calories daily between ages 2 and 3; 1,200–1,800 calories daily for girls and 1,200–2,000 kcals for boys between ages 4 and 8; 1,400–2,200 calories for girls and 1,600–2,600 calories for boys between ages 9 and 13; and 1,800–2,400 calories for girls and 2,000–3,200 calories for boys between ages 14 and 18.

Protein needs are also increased during periods of growth, especially during the first year of life and during growth spurts. The importance of protein was discussed in Question 18. Protein needs may not be met when animal foods are eliminated, as they are the primary source of protein for most Americans. General guidelines estimate that children require between two and four ounces of protein daily between ages 2 and 3; three to five ounces daily for girls and three to five and one-half ounces for boys between ages 4 and 8; four to six ounces for girls and five to six and one-half ounces for boys between ages 9 and 13; and five to six and one-half ounces for girls and five and one-half to seven ounces for boys between ages 14 and 18. Vegetarian and vegan diets can often be suboptimal in total daily calories and protein if not planned with care or food choices are high in nonnutritive calories, sugar, and unhealthy fat.

Beside calorie and protein needs, as during pregnancy, specific nutrients are increased during periods of growth. Calcium needs are increased to support bone and tooth development and growth. Since most calcium is found in dairy foods, care must be taken to adequately supplement a plant-based diet in calcium for children. Children ages 1–3 require 700 milligrams of calcium daily; ages 4–8 require 1,000 milligrams daily; and ages 9–18 require 1,300 milligrams daily. Vitamin D requirements are also increased to support the growth of strong bones. Babies and children need at least 400 International Units (IU) of vitamin D daily. Getting daily sun exposure also helps to increase vitamin D levels.

All B vitamin needs increase during growth because they are important for metabolism, energy, and heart and nervous system health. Children eating a plant-based diet must pay particular attention to vitamin B_{12} food sources and supplements because most food sources of vitamin B_{12} are found in animal foods, such as eggs, fish, meat, and poultry. Babies require 0.5 micrograms of vitamin B_{12} daily; toddlers require 1.6 micrograms; ages 4–8 require 1.2 micrograms; ages 9–13 require 1.8 micrograms; and teens require 2.4 micrograms. Pregnant teenage girls require 2.6 micrograms.

Vitamin E is one nutrient that strengthens the immune system and works as an antioxidant. Antioxidants help to slow down environmental processes that damage body cells and contribute to the aging process and disease. Adequate daily vitamin E also supports healthy cardiovascular health and metabolic processes. Food sources of vitamin E include vegetable oils and nuts and seeds. This is one nutrient easily supplied with a plant-based diet. However, someone with food allergies (discussed in Question 22) may have suboptimal intakes and require a dietary supplement to meet their needs. Ages 1–3 require nine IU of vitamin E daily; ages 4–8 need 10.4 IU; ages 9–13 need 16.4 IU; and teens need 22 IU daily.

Iron is another critical nutrient that increases during growth periods, especially for girls when they begin menstruation. The importance of iron was discussed in Question 20. Children require 7–10 milligrams of iron daily. During their teens, boys need an estimated 11 milligrams a day while girls require 15 milligrams daily. Because iron is found in meat and other animal foods, special care must be taken to provide adequate sources of iron in the diet.

Questions 18, and 19 discussed each of these critical nutrients, their importance, and plant-based food sources in depth. With careful menu planning, and dietary supplementation when indicated, children can grow properly and remain healthy following a plant-based diet.

22. Can those with food allergies follow a plant-based diet?

Yes, they can. For anyone who experiences a negative reaction after eating a food, eating a plant-based diet is really no different from eating a meat-based diet. The individual must always be aware of what they are eating and of added ingredients to any food they eat. In addition, they must plan their diets carefully to replace any nutrients that are eaten in suboptimal amounts because entire food groups may be eliminated either due to an adverse food reaction or due to exclusion of animal foods. Whenever an entire food group is eliminated, nutrient deficiencies can occur if the diet is not planned correctly to replace nutrients found in the eliminated food(s) via other foods or dietary supplements.

Food allergies always involve the immune system. The job of the immune system is to protect the body from foreign invaders that have the potential to cause a serious illness or death. A food allergy is thought to occur when the immune system mistakenly identifies a specific food as a threat and over reacts by attacking it. It is estimated that 90 percent of food allergies worldwide are to eggs, cow's milk, legumes (beans, peanuts), sesame seeds, shellfish, soy, tree nuts, and wheat. However, any food has the potential to cause an allergic reaction for some people. It is still unclear why a person develops a food allergy. There are many theories why a person becomes allergic to food, ranging from being "too clean" as a society, birth methods, lack of exposure to a food when young, vaccines, and genetics. Allergic reactions to a food range from minor, such as runny nose, hives, or upset stomach, to severe and life threatening, such as anaphylaxis.

Less threatening, but still life altering, are food sensitivities and intolerances. Many people believe that all negative reactions to a food are a food allergy. But not all negative reactions to a food are an allergic response. The distinction between a food intolerance and a food allergy is that true food allergies involve the immune system and are usually life threatening. Food intolerances do not involve the immune system, are generally not life threatening, and almost always affect the digestive system. Symptoms of a food intolerance vary from person to person. The most frequently reported symptoms include abdominal pain or stomachache, bloating, constipation or diarrhea, cough, gas, headaches or migraines, hives, irritable bowel, and runny nose. Symptoms begin anywhere from within a few minutes to a few hours after eating a food that triggers the reaction.

Food sensitivity reactions differ from food allergies and food intolerances. These negative reactions sometimes involve the immune system but may also affect the brain, gastrointestinal system, joints, skin, and respiratory tract. Food sensitivities tend to be much more complicated to diagnose because symptoms often seem unrelated to a specific food or may occur when specific foods are eaten together. Symptoms can also occur days and weeks after eating the suspected food. Food sensitivity reactions are difficult to diagnose and range from minor symptoms to debilitating to life threatening. Food sensitivity symptoms, as with food intolerances, vary from person to person and include all the same symptoms that can occur with food allergies and intolerances. However, many unrelated symptoms associated with chronic diseases or conditions are also thought to indicate a food sensitivity reaction. These include arthritis, autism, inflammatory bowel disease, joint pain, "brain fog" or memory loss, nutritional deficiencies, and numerous environmental allergies.

The most common food allergens found in a plant-based diet are to eggs, fish and seafood, legumes and peanuts, milk, sesame seeds, soy, tree nuts, and wheat. Specific fruits and vegetables may also cause an allergic reaction and will be specific from person to person. Food intolerances are most often associated with decreasing amounts of digestive enzyme production in the body, which usually decreases with age or a chronic health condition. In some people genetics may prevent enzyme production, which can decrease an individual's ability to digest foods. Some foods also have specific compounds, such as amines found in protein foods, that when digested may produce a negative reaction. All of these factors can lead to a food intolerance. While any food can produce an intolerance reaction, the most common food intolerances are to fructose and lactose, which are found in fruit, honey, and milk.

Nickel allergies are becoming increasingly diagnosed as more and more people eat a plant-based diet because foods that are a staple of plant-based diets are often high in nickel content. Nickel is a metal commonly found in the environment and foods. Common items, such as jewelry, coins, keys, cell phones, eyeglass frames, paper clips, pens, orthodontic braces, stainless steel cooking and eating utensils, and clothing buttons, belts, and zippers contain nickel. Foods that are found to be high in nickel include black tea, nuts and seeds, soy, oats, buckwheat, whole wheat, wheat germ, whole wheat pasta, multigrain breads and cereals, and legumes (chick peas, lentils, peas, peanuts, soy, tofu). Fruits with high levels of nickel include bananas, pears, and all canned fruits. Many vegetables are also good sources of nickel, particularly asparagus, broccoli, brussels sprouts, cauliflower, spinach, and all canned vegetables. Symptoms of a nickel allergy include skin rash, itching, or blisters that can progress to more severe symptoms such as asthma, bleeding gums, and respiratory problems. Those with a nickel allergy must avoid all foods that contain even low amounts of nickel and may even need to incorporate some animal foods into their diet to remain healthy because alternatives to animal-based foods are often high in nickel.

23. How does someone who has gastrointestinal disease follow a plant-based diet?

Eating a plant-based diet can be tricky for someone who has a disorder or disease of the gastrointestinal tract. There are many abnormal reactions to food that include the gastrointestinal system. The most widely diagnosed are Celiac and Crohn's disease, food-dependent exercise-induced anaphylaxis, food-induced enterocolitis syndrome, food protein-induced proctocolitis, oral allergy syndrome, sulfite induced asthma, small intestinal bacterial overgrowth (SIBO), and leaky gut syndrome. While many plant-based diets may be difficult to follow for individuals that have a gastrointestinal disease, proper meal preparation, moderate consumption of plant foods, and avoidance of trigger plant foods can avoid negative health consequences.

Celiac disease is an autoimmune disease. Celiacs are allergic to gluten, a protein found in barley, rye, and wheat. Gluten can trigger an immune reaction that damages the small intestine. This leads to decreased absorption of nutrients and malnutrition. Successful treatment requires a strict gluten free diet. Gluten is found in any food that has barley, rye, and wheat as an ingredient, such as pasta and noodles, baked breads and pastries, crackers, cereals and granola, pancakes, waffles, French toast, biscuits, panko breadcrumbs, stuffing, dressings, sauces, gravies, flour tortillas, beers and wines, and brewers' yeast. Those who eat plant-based diets often eat many foods made from these grains. But there are many gluten free alternatives for celiac patients that also provide similar nutritional value. These are corn, chickpeas, oats, rice and flours made from almonds, amaranth, arrowroot, buckwheat, cassava, corn, chickpea, coconut, oats, brown rice, sorghum, tapioca, and teff. Quinoa, a popular grain that is eaten in many plant-based diets, is thought to be gluten free. However, it is considered to be at high risk for contamination with wheat, barley, and rye. Celiac patients are advised to eliminate it from their diet.

Crohn's disease is an inflammatory bowel disease that causes inflammation of the digestive tract. While symptoms are similar to celiac disease, food is not thought to trigger it. However, raw fruits and vegetables often aggravate symptoms and must be eliminated or cooked thoroughly for tolerance. Sometimes elimination of gluten is also helpful in mitigating symptoms.

Food-dependent exercise-induced anaphylaxis (FDEIA) is a rare disorder that occurs only if an individual eats a specific food and exercises within a one to four-hour period of time before or after eating it. Alcohol, apples, celery, dairy, eggs, fish, fruit, legumes, milk, nuts, shellfish, and wheat are the most common trigger foods of FDEIA. Why this reaction occurs is still unknown.

Food protein-induced enterocolitis syndrome (FPIES) commonly occurs in infants and children, but can occur in adults. Chicken, eggs, cow's milk, nuts, peanuts, rice, soy, turkey, and wheat are the most common trigger foods that cause the symptoms of severe and repetitive vomiting along with diarrhea, lethargy, and poor growth.

Food protein-induced proctocolitis (FPIPC) usually occurs in infants and is triggered by cow's milk or soy protein, although corn and eggs have been known to cause symptoms.

Proteins found in environmental pollens may also trigger oral allergy syndrome. These same proteins are also found in some fruits and vegetables. When these foods are eaten in their raw form, susceptible individuals have an allergic reaction. However, if these foods are cooked, the protein is broken down, and the individual is frequently able to eat it without symptoms.

Sulfite-induced asthma is a reaction to sulfites found in foods. Sulfites are often found naturally in broccoli, cabbage, cauliflower, chives, eggs, garlic, kale, leeks, onions, peanuts, black tea, vinegar and other fermented foods. But they are frequently added as a preservative to foods, such as alcoholic drinks, baked goods, shredded coconut, condiments, fruits, canned or bottled fruit and vegetables, gelatin and pudding or filling mixes, dried fruits and snacks, drink mixes, grains, jams and preserves, molasses, pastries, soup mixes, and vegetables.

Leaky gut syndrome, also known as increased intestinal permeability, is thought to have a negative effect on health. Leaky gut occurs when undigested foods, bacteria, and toxins are able to pass through a normally tight gastrointestinal epithelial cell barrier into the blood stream through "holes" created by damage from a chronic disease or food sensitivity. This in turn leads to other symptoms. Any food may increase this damage to the GI system and requires the use of an elimination diet to determine the cause.

Small intestinal bacterial overgrowth (SIBO), or dysbiosis, is associated with an imbalance of bacteria in the small intestine. The small and large intestines contain large numbers of bacteria that are essential for good health and digestion. This bacterial environment is known as the microbiome (discussed in Question 11). When bacterial balance is disrupted, either due to diet, disease, or food sensitivities, symptoms can occur. Treatment with probiotics or fermented foods and a gluten and/or dairy free diet are the usual treatment options to restore gut health and integrity. Those with small intestinal bacterial overgrowth (SIBO) must also avoid foods high in FODMAPs (fermentable oligosaccharides, disaccharides, monosaccharides, and polyols), which are carbohydrate foods that may produce symptoms in susceptible individuals. High amounts of FODMAPs are found in apples, garlic, some fruits, high fructose corn syrup, honey, legumes, milk, onion, rye, some vegetables, and wheat.

In addition to these food sensitivities, plant foods also have naturally occurring phytochemicals, known as antinutrients (discussed in-depth in Question 9). These antinutrients discourage animals, fungi, insects, and humans from eating them because they often have a bitter taste or cause gastrointestinal upset. Some of these compounds can be toxic. For example, the seeds of corn, oats, rice, and wheat are considered grains. Hazelnuts, pecans, and walnuts are the seeds of trees. Legumes, such as chickpeas, lentils, peas, peanuts, and soybeans, are the seeds of beans. Exposure to these seeds can cause intestinal lining damage to whoever eats them. This in turn may cause inflammation and malabsorption of nutrients and gastrointestinal distress. Some of these toxins are also thought to be the root cause of allergies, autoimmune diseases, food intolerances or sensitivities, and other chronic illnesses in humans who cannot tolerate them. For example, undercooked beans can cause digestive problems because they have a compound called aflatoxin, which ferments in the gastrointestinal tract if inadequately digested. Aflatoxins are chemicals produced by specific molds that grow in soil, decaying vegetation, hay, and grains. Aflatoxins are found naturally in peanuts, beans and lentils, pistachios, cereals that contain raw seeds and nuts, maize, some dried fruits and figs, black pepper, chilies, and spices. Foods considered to be a high risk for aflatoxins are extremely toxic and carcinogenic and may cause death. Most countries strictly regulate these foods. Legumes, such as peanuts, and other risky foods are inspected for mold and eliminated from the food supply or chemically decontaminated. Cooking beans properly, which does not completely eliminate aflatoxins, will usually breakdown the legume structure and reduce the toxic effect enough that an individual is able to digest it properly. Most sensitive individuals are often able to eat fully cooked beans without symptoms.

24. Are all vegetarian and vegan foods healthy and good for you?

Individuals who follow a plant-based diet often select processed foods to eat, such as meat alternatives, crackers, and cookies. A food is considered processed if the natural form of that food undergoes any method that turns it into a food product. Methods include chopping, cooking, curing, drying, fermenting, freezing, heating, washing, packaging, pasteurizing, pickling, smoking, and/or adding ingredients to extend shelf life or to change the flavor. Unprocessed fruits, grains, nuts, seeds, and vegetables are foods found in their natural form. They are usually healthy food choices when eaten in moderation. However, not all vegan or vegetarian foods are healthy food products because of their added ingredients and preservatives. Choosing a healthy carbohydrate processed food is important for everyone, not just those on a plant-based diet. These foods have notoriously unhealthy amounts of added fat, sugar, and salt to improve their acceptance. Taste matters, and if a food does not taste good, people will not eat it or buy it.

However, meat alternatives are more complex than processed carbohydrate choices when looking at nutritional value. Meat alternatives are considered to be a meatless food that has the same taste, appearance, texture, and nutritional value of an animal protein source that is not processed. Question 17 briefly looked at the ingredients and nutrition comparison between traditional meat alternatives, such as a NEAT burger, and current-day meat alternatives, such as Beyond Meat burgers. This comparison showed that the ingredients and nutrition quality between these two versions of plant-based meats varied greatly.

For many years, meat alternative choices were limited because few people ate plant-based meats. Vegans and vegetarians relied on soy products, such as miso, tofu, tempeh, soy nuts, and soymilk, along with legumes, nuts, seeds, and yuba to meet daily protein needs. Processed meatless protein products, known as meat analogues, first became available in 1899. The first commercially available meat analogue, Nutfoda, was offered to the public in 1911. The Soy Burger, produced by Madison Foods of Tennessee, was brought to market in 1937. Meat analogues continued to evolve, becoming more popular during the 1960s and 1970s after *Diet for a Small Planet* by Frances Moore Lappé was published. At that time, meat analogues were made mostly from canola oil, sunflower seeds, wheat gluten, nuts, soybeans, and yuba. But in 1972, food scientists perfected the method of making a vegetable protein from peas. Using a milling process, raw peas were separated into starch and protein components. The protein component was then bound together into laminated sheets. When water was added to these laminated sheets, they could be molded and shaped to resemble a piece of meat. Soy protein isolates and concentrates were further developed into textured soy proteins that also increased the variety and protein content of meat alternatives. Popular meat analogues at that time included Tofurky (alternate for turkey), FriChik (alternative for fried chicken), Choplets (alternative for pork chops), Soyloin steaks (alternative for sirloin), Vegelinks (alternative for sausage links), Vegetable Skallops, Stripples (alternative for bacon), Mock chicken Tempeh Salad, Tofu Wieners (alternative to hot dogs), and numerous meatless burger brands (NEAT burger and Back Yard Burgers, to name a few). After "The China Study" by T. Colin Campbell was published in 2016 (discussed in Question 12), a resurgence of interest and demand for meat alternatives occurred. In recent years the evolution of meat alternatives produced the increasingly popular Impossible Burger and Beyond Burger brands offered in 2019. Many restaurants and fast-food chains have added them to their menus, and even more products are becoming available, such as plant-based chicken and bacon products. These burgers claim to look, taste, and "bleed" like real meat. But nutritionally they are much different from past meat analogues.

Nutrition and public health researchers and the Food and Agriculture Organization of the United Nations use the NOVA classification system to "categorize foods according to the extent and purpose of food processing, rather than in terms of nutrients." The NOVA system classifies all foods and food products into four distinct groupings: unprocessed or minimally processed foods, processed culinary ingredients, processed foods, and ultra-processed food and drink products. According to the NOVA classification system, both the Impossible Burger and Beyond Burger are considered ultraprocessed food products, meaning they either use food substances rarely used in kitchens (such as hydrolyzed proteins and protein isolates) and/or use additives (colors, emulsifiers, thickeners) to make the final product more palatable and appealing.

The ingredients for these two meatless burgers appear in Table 3.

But how do these food products compare to each other and real meat nutritionally? The nutrition facts for a grilled hamburger, Impossible Burger, and Beyond Burger appear in Table 4.

The meat alternative burgers appear to offer the same amount of protein as animal meat, but they are higher in calories, fat, saturated fat, and

Table 3 Ingredients for two meatless burger brands

Impossible Burger	Beyond Burger
Water, soy protein concentrated, coconut oil, sunflower oil, natural flavors, 2% or less of: potato protein, methylcellulose, yeast extract, cultured dextrose, food starch modified, soy leghemoglobin, salt, soy protein isolate, mixed tocopherols, zinc gluconate, thiamine hydrochloride, sodium ascorbate, niacin, pyridoxine hydrochloride, riboflavin, vitamin B$_{12}$	Water, pea protein isolate, expeller-pressed canola oil, refined coconut oil, rice protein, natural flavors, cocoa butter, mung bean protein, methylcellulose, potato starch, apple extract, salt, potassium chloride, vinegar, lemon juice concentrate, sunflower lecithin, pomegranate fruit powder, beet juice extract

Table 4 Burger nutrition facts

Per single burger (No bun)	4 oz Lean beef grilled hamburger	4 oz Impossible Burger	4 oz Beyond Burger
Calories	170	240	260
Protein (gram)	23 (3 ounces)	19 (2.5 ounces)	20 (2.75 ounces)
Fats (gram)	8	14	18
Saturated fat (gram)	3.5	8	5
Carbohydrates (gram)	0	9	5
Sodium (milligram)	75	370	350
Cholesterol (milligram)	69	0	0

sodium. Animal protein foods are also composed of all essential amino acids necessary for good health, while plant proteins are not. Question 19 discussed protein quality in depth and the ways plant proteins need to be combined with other foods to complete their amino acid profile. In addition to this concern, the FAO raises concerns about ultra-processed food products. These foods use chemically manufactured ingredients not found naturally, are nutritionally imbalanced, replace whole foods in the diet, are aggressively marketed without accurately informing the consumer of their manufacturing process (organic and non-GMO ingredients are not always used as many consumers assume), and are in general associated with increased rates of obesity and chronic diseases and all-cause mortality.

Dr. Kara Fitzgerald, a functional medicine physician, highlights the questionable nutrition composition of many of these "faux meats" in her 2019 article "Faux Meats: Good for the Planet—but What about Your Health?" Bottom line: reading food labels of all processed plant-based foods, not just meat alternatives, and picking minimally processed plant foods is essential when making wise nutrition choices for anyone eating a plant-based diet.

25. Why is soy so controversial, and is it bad for health?

Soy is a very controversial plant-based food. Some in the health community feel soy is beneficial and protective, mitigating symptoms of osteoporosis, menopause (hot flashes), and protective against hormonal cancers (breast and prostate cancers). Others feel it may actually increase the risk for breast cancer, dementia, and thyroid disease. In addition to these concerns, those allergic to soy and nickel (soy is a good source of nickel) may be adversely affected by soy in the diet (discussed in Question 22). To date, no clear consensus has been reached about the health benefits of soy.

Soy is a plant species found within the legume family. Legumes are the third largest family of flowering plants in the world and have over 20,000 different species. The terms beans, legumes, and pulses are used interchangeably to describe these plants, but there is a difference between a pulse and legumes and beans. Legumes and beans (black beans, chickpeas, kidney beans, lentils, navy beans, peas, pinto beans, etc.) are plants that have a pod. A pulse is the dry, edible seed of a legume plant. For example, a pea pod is considered a legume, but the pea inside the pod is called a pulse. Soybeans, while part of the legume family, are not considered a pulse because they have high amounts of oil that make them moist and not dry like most edible seeds.

Soybeans are good sources of protein, B vitamins, folate, fiber, iron, magnesium, phosphorus, potassium, and polyunsaturated and monoun-saturated fatty acids. Soy is often used as a meat alternative because it is a complete protein that contains all nine essential amino acids found in animal foods. These nutritional qualities make them a highly desir-able food choice when eating a plant-based diet. Soy is classified into fermented or unfermented forms. Fermented soy are foods that have been processed with beneficial bacteria, mold, or yeast, which is thought to improve digestibility and maintain a health gastrointestinal microbiome. Fermented soy foods include miso, natto, soy sauce, and tempeh. Unfer-mented soy foods include edamame, soy cheese and milk, dry roasted and boiled soybeans, soy-based veggie burgers, and tofu. There are also pro-cessed versions of soy, such as soy protein powder and meal replacement bars that add soy isoflavones.

Soy is unique because it has a high concentration of the isoflavones genistein and daidzein. Isoflavones are a type of plant estrogen that mim-ics the hormone estrogen normally made in the human body. This estro-genic effect, which is weaker than estrogen the body produces naturally, is a source of controversy because studies are conflicting on whether these isoflavones are beneficial or harmful. Because of this, some clinicians advise soy should be avoided, especially if someone has a history of breast or prostate cancer.

Clinical research into the health benefits of soy protein increased after a 1995 meta-analysis of 38 clinical studies showed that consumption of an estimated 50 grams of soy protein a day (equivalent to 1½ pounds of tofu or eight 8-ounce glasses of soy milk) instead of animal protein reduced harmful cholesterol levels by almost 13 percent. This reduction of blood cholesterol levels was estimated to reduce the risk for heart attacks, stroke, and other cardiovascular diseases by greater than 20 per-cent. But a comprehensive research study by the nutrition committee of the American Heart Association in 2000 found that eating 50 grams of soy protein only lowered cardiovascular risk by 3 percent. The U.S. FDA reviewed additional scientific studies in 2017 and proposed revoking the 1995 claim of soy proteins health benefits due to inconsistent findings. Soy protein is still considered a healthy choice, however, if it reduces or replaces red meats, which have been associated with an increased risk for cardiovascular disease.

Including soy in the diet has also gained support with postmenopausal women to help reduce menopausal symptoms. It is estimated that 70–80 percent of women in the United States experience perimenopausal and menopausal symptoms of hot flashes and weight gain. Because soy is a phytoestrogen, it has been used as an alternative form of hormone replacement therapy to reduce these unpleasant symptoms. Traditional long-term hormone therapies are associated with an increased risk for breast cancer and stroke. Women in Asian countries who eat soy daily have levels of the isoflavone genistein 12 times higher than American women and experience much lower rates of menopausal symptoms. However, research has not confirmed that soy is the primary factor contributing to these lower rates. In theory, it is thought that the phytoestrogen effect of soy isoflavones provides an estrogen boost as natural estrogen levels decline. But several meta analyses by the AHA and a study reported in the *Journal of the American Medical Association* (*JAMA*) in 2006 and a 2013 review of 43 controlled trials concluded there was not enough evidence to support this theory and more research was warranted.

The effect of soy on hormonal cancers is also very controversial. Although soy is associated with mimicking estrogen, there is a theory that soy can block the effects of estrogen as well and possibly reduce the risk for breast or prostate cancers. But there is also a belief that soy may actually stimulate cancer growth. Some research studies find that high doses of isoflavones or isolated soy protein extracts stimulate breast cancer growth. However, studies that observed human consumption of soy foods found that soy had a protective or neutral effect. The Shanghai Women's Health Study followed 73,223 Chinese women for more than seven years and is considered the most detailed study of breast cancer risk in a population with a high soy dietary consumption. Study results showed that women who consumed the most soy foods in their daily diet, equivalent to an estimated average of 46 milligrams of soy isoflavones, had a 59 percent lower risk for premenopausal breast cancer. This study also found that breast cancer risk was reduced by 43 percent when soy foods were introduced into the diet during adolescence. The Breast Cancer Family Registry is another study that investigated the soy isoflavone intake of 6,235 women diagnosed with breast cancer in the United States and Canada. This study found that women who ate the highest amounts of soy isoflavones had a 21 percent lower risk of death compared to those who consumed low amounts of them.

In men, prostate cancer incidence is the highest in Western countries and the lowest in Asian countries. Research finds that Chinese and Japanese men who moved to Western countries increased their risk for prostate cancer. Genistein and daidzein is found to collect in the male prostate and thought to act as a weak estrogen that is protective against cancer. Studies find that unfermented soy and total soy food amounts can reduce prostate cancer risk. However, not all studies verify these findings and continued research in this area is needed.

There have also been some studies that theorize soy isoflavones, such as daidzein, may reduce memory and cognition declines that occur as a person ages. Again, there has been no clear scientific evidence that proves this theory. A review of 13 studies concluded that approximately 50 percent of these studies found supplementing with isoflavones improved cognition in older men and women, including improvements in memory, attention, and information processing speed. However, the other 50 percent found no differences and one large study of men found soy actually decreased cognitive functioning. Continued research is needed as to the effect soy may have on aging.

The last concern about soy is its effect on the thyroid gland. The thyroid is found in the front part of the neck below the Adam's apple. It is responsible for secreting different hormones that influence metabolism, growth and development, and body temperature. Thyroid hormones are also critical for brain development during pregnancy, infancy, and childhood. In one small study, 60 patients who had subclinical hypothyroidism (a mild form of a sluggish thyroid) were given either a placebo or a supplement that contained 30 grams of soy protein (approximately what one might eat on a vegetarian meal plan). Researchers found that women who took the soy supplements had a greater risk for developing clinical hypothyroidism (symptoms that required thyroid replacement medication) than those who received the placebo. However, they also found that those who took the soy supplement also had a greater reduction in insulin resistance, inflammatory markers, and blood pressure. This is one area that continues to need more research.

There are many unanswered questions and conflicting data about the health benefits of soy and much more research is needed. But it does appear that food sources of soy, such as edamame, miso, soy milk and nuts, tempeh, and tofu, are safe when consumed from organic sources and in moderate amounts. Those with breast or prostate cancers are advised to limit organic soy consumption to no more than two servings a day until more research is available.

26. What are lectins, and are they a problem when eating a vegetarian or vegan diet?

Lectins, also called glycoproteins, are proteins that bind to carbohydrates. Lectins are found in beans, pulses, grains, some fruits and vegetables, nuts, coffee, chocolate, and some herbs and spices (marjoram, nutmeg, peppermint). Pulses and grains have the highest concentrations of lectins and lectins are a natural insecticide plants use to protect it from insects, disease, and consumption by animals.

As discussed in Questions 9 and 23, plants have compounds known as antinutrients that discourage animals and humans from eating them. These antinutrients often have a bitter taste and can cause unpleasant gastrointestinal symptoms as well as block the absorption of nutrients from food. Animals are unable to efficiently digest lectins, which bind to the gastrointestinal cells in animals. This in turn produces gastrointestinal distress that usually ensures the animal will not eat it again. Research finds that compounds found in lectins, especially when eaten raw, can bind to the cells in the digestive tract. This in turn negatively affects the gastrointestinal flora (microbiome), which in turn affects nutrient absorption. Because lectins bind to cells for prolonged periods of time, it is thought that this may initiate an autoimmune reaction possibly triggering chronic illnesses, such as allergies or sensitivities, autoimmune diseases, cancer, leaky gut, rheumatoid arthritis, and type I diabetes. Continued research is needed in this area to verify these theories.

Many lectins in vegetables (chickpeas, tomatoes, legumes, peas, fava beans) are nontoxic. Lectins are found in the greatest amounts in raw legumes (beans, lentils, peas, soybeans, and peanuts) and whole grains (wheat). But they are also found in vegetables. Rich sources of lectins include potatoes, eggplant, peppers, wheat germ, and tomatoes. Lectins that are cooked before eating are usually denatured enough to be eaten without symptoms. For example, raw or undercooked kidney beans contain the lectin phytohemagglutinin and are toxic when eaten uncooked. This lectin can cause red blood cells to clump together leading to symptoms of lectin poisoning. Acute symptoms of lectin poisoning include diarrhea, nausea, and vomiting. Other symptoms include bloating, gas, stomach upset, and weight loss. However, well-cooked kidney beans (soaked for five hours in water and cooked for at least one hour) are rendered safe to eat because the cooking process destroys most of the lectin in a food, reducing its ability to bind to gastrointestinal cells or other compounds in foods. However, eating large quantities of any legume will often produce gas and bloating. This happens because legumes are difficult to digest by humans because they contain the resistant starch oligosaccharide. Thus, undigested legumes in the gastrointestinal tract are fermented by microbiome bacteria, which then produce the symptoms of bloating and gas. Lectins also contain gluten, which is problematic for anyone with Celiac or Crohn's disease or gluten intolerance.

Lectins, however, also have positive health benefits. We know lectins play a role in cell interactions and immune regulation. Some research finds that their antimicrobial properties are effective against some infections, such as staph and E. coli, and may even block the growth of fungus responsible for yeast infections. They are also an excellent source of protein, making them a favorite animal protein replacement choice for those following a plant-based diet. Lectins have been found to lower colorectal cancer and may improve diabetes and promote weight loss. Research also shows they can lower inflammation.

So, should someone eating a plant-based diet avoid lectins? The best advice given by most integrative practitioners is that lectins should always be eaten well cooked and infrequently. Because some lectins are temperature sensitive, they are best cooked using a pressure cooker. Beans should be soaked well before cooking, changing the water frequently during the soaking process. Soy should be organic and fermented. Breads and cereals made from sprouted seeds usually have lower amounts of lectin, except for alfalfa, which actually increases in lectin when sprouted. It is recommended that eating the seeds and peels of these foods should be avoided because they have the highest lectin concentration. Conventional cooking methods destroys lectins and renders them safe to eat. Nutritionfacts .org has very informative videos about lectins and how to cook them.

The popular book *The Plant Paradox: The Hidden Dangers in "Healthy" Foods That Cause Disease and Weight Gain* by Dr. Steven Gundry was published in 2017 and promotes a lectin-free diet. Dr. Gundry theorizes that lectin-containing foods actually are toxic to the body, promoting inflammation that can cause weight gain and health problems. But research about this theory does not support his thesis. A 2004 review in the journal *Toxicon* found that cooking foods high in lectin substantially lowered any negative health effects they might have on the body. In 2016, a review in the journal *Current Protein & Peptide Science* concluded that the anticancer activity found in mushrooms indicates that lectin may have a possible role in cancer treatment of tumors. Given the strong research evidence that support the positive health impacts of fruits, nuts, pulses, and vegetables that often contain lectin, it appears their health benefits far outweigh any negative consequences they might have.

Life as a Vegetarian or Vegan

27. How do I transition to a plant-based diet?

It is not difficult to transition to eating a plant-based diet, but it does require some soul searching, planning, and gradual implementation to be successful. When deciding if a plant-based diet is appropriate, the first question an individual should ask themselves is why they wish to eliminate meat or animal foods from their diet. For instance, is it for health, religious, or environmental reasons or to support the ethical treatment of animals, or all of these? Answering this question focuses the person on their motivation for eliminating animal foods and allows them to further decide which plant-based diet is best for their beliefs, goals, and lifestyle, that is, flexitarian, pescatarian, semivegetarian, vegetarian, vegan, or whole food plant.

The most common mistake people make when eliminating animal foods is improperly balancing their diet nutritionally, which can result in potential nutrient deficiencies (discussed in Questions 9 and 19). Becoming educated about nutrition and how to plan a realistic diet that is nutritionally balanced to meet daily nutrition requirements and replace nutrients found in animal foods is essential when transitioning to a plant-based diet. Another common mistake people make is to eat a meal plan of only vegetables, which results in becoming full quickly and eating less calories and nutrients than needed. Feelings of hunger, fatigue, and unintended weight loss can be the result. For some people, transitioning to a diet without animal foods can be challenging and intimidating psychologically. Besides the tie to eating disorders and depression, discussed in Question 9, some people have a very difficult time feeling satisfied or properly nourished when animal foods are eliminated. Eating meat as part of the diet is a strongly established custom in many cultures and often associated with health, power, and wealth. Meat is also an integral custom for many religious and cultural holidays and celebrations.

It is usually recommended that individuals gradually transition their way of eating over a one-month period. Moderate diet changes are less intimidating and not as overwhelming, which helps to ensure long-term success. Another benefit to a slow transition is increasing gastrointestinal tolerance to a plant-based diet. Plant-based diets are much higher in dietary fiber than most animal-based diets. A gradual transition allows the body to adapt to increased amounts of fiber, which helps the digestive system adjust gradually to avoid uncomfortable and unpleasant gastrointestinal symptoms that can occur when fiber is increased (discussed in Question 9). Eliminating animal foods also changes how people grocery shop and cook, the restaurants they go to when dining out, and interactions with family and friends, especially during holidays. New habits need to be made. Gradual transitioning allows time to learn new recipes and food preparation methods that take time to adjust to. Favorite restaurants may not be "plant" friendly and so it may mean leaving behind preferred restaurants and finding new ones. Gradual transitioning can also encourage family and friends, who may not accept or be supportive of the diet, to become familiar and more accepting of their loved ones change in eating habits.

Luckily, there are a number of cookbooks and recipe websites that have a plethora of plant-based recipes that make transitioning to a plant-based menu much easier than in the past. Learning to read and interpret food labels is an important skill to also have when grocery shopping so that wise nutrition choices are made and purchasing processed plant foods high in unhealthy amounts of saturated fats, sodium, and sugars avoided. Label reading is discussed in Question 29. As plant-based diets become more popular and meat alternatives become increasingly available, restaurants are much more accommodating and family and friends more accepting.

Nutrition guidelines are available to help an individual transition to a healthy plant-based diet. Since 1916, the U.S. Department of Agriculture (USDA) has published a Food Guide to help Americans eat healthy. Over the years it has been updated to the most recent 2005 MyPyramid Food Guidance System for Americans. Recommended dietary guideline are presented by food group, which includes animal foods, in a food pyramid graphic that highlights groups of food and recommended serving sizes that ensures good health for the majority of healthy people. In 2011, the MyPlate was introduced, changing the pyramid into a plate with a food portion graphic that is easier to understand for consumers. Vegetarians and vegans also have their own Food Pyramid and MyPlate graphics and guidelines to help them eat a balanced diet that will help prevent nutrition deficiencies.

General guidelines for both vegan and vegetarian adults recommend the daily food guides for six basic food groups listed in Table 5 (herbs and spices are not considered a food group but are included because they provide phytonutrients that are beneficial for health).

These guidelines, along with other published protocols by the International Vegan Association and Physicians Committee for Responsible Medicine, provide excellent guidance along with recipes to assist people during their transition from an animal-based diet to a plant-based one.

Table 5   Plant-Based Nutrition Guidelines for six basic food groups

Food group	Serving size	Number of daily servings
Fruit	½ cup fresh, canned, frozen; juice ¼ cup dried	3 to 4
Beans, peas, lentils, soy	½ cup cooked beans, peas, lentils ½ cup tofu 8 ounces soy milk	3 to 6
Herbs, spices	fresh or dried	liberal use
Nuts, peanuts, peanut butter, seeds, nut butters	¼ cup nuts/seeds 2 tablespoons nut butters	1 to 3
Plant oils	1 teaspoon	up to 5
Vegetables	½ cup cooked 1 cup raw	4 to 6
Whole grains	1 slice bread 1 cup cereal ½ cup cooked rice, pasta, other whole grains	4 to 6

28. Is it difficult to eat out in restaurants or in public places when following a vegetarian or vegan diet?

It can be challenging to eat out when following a plant-based diet. However, as plant-based diets become more popular restaurants are increasingly offering meat alternatives on their menus and will often accommodate requests for plant-based entrées. For those who have transitioned to a plant-based diet, the best strategy when eating out is to plan ahead. Most restaurants post an online menu. Researching a restaurant website before dining there can help determine if the menu can provide a satisfying meal. If menu options are limited, combining different à la carte menu offerings may the most sensible way to put together a plant-based meal, such as a salad with added chickpeas, side of potato or rice, and a cooked vegetable or vegetable chili with a baked potato and steamed vegetable. If it is known that plant-based protein menu options are limited, eating a small snack before going to the restaurant can also prevent hunger and supply any missing nutrients from the meal that the restaurant cannot accommodate. Restaurants are increasingly willing to honor special requests when dining out during slow times and off-peak hours. Calling the restaurant before going can also sometimes allow them to accommodate plant-based meal requests prior to arrival. But it also important to realize that if the meal is not well-balanced due to the lack of meatless options, missing protein at one meal will not cause nutritional harm over the long-term. There are also a number of smartphone apps available that research various restaurants, providing reviews and recommendations. The HappyCow identifies restaurants state-by-state that are vegan and vegetarian friendly. Vegan.com also offers a review and listing of restaurants that offer vegan meals.

Chinese, Greek, Indian, Italian, Japanese, and Mexican restaurants offer the most plant-based selections on their menus that can be either vegetarian or vegan. Chinese, Thai, and Vietnamese restaurants include stir-fried vegetable dishes, tofu and vegetable dishes, steamed rice, vegetarian spring rolls, and vegetarian noodle soups on their menus. Greek restaurants include tahini, hummus, pita bread, vegetable dolmades, Greek salad, roasted eggplant, grilled vegetables or wraps in their meal selections. Indian restaurants include many tomato-based chickpea lentil and vegetable curries, dal, roti, pickles and chutneys, and rice. Italian restaurants include vegetarian pizza without cheese, pasta dishes with fresh vegetables, tomato and basil bruschetta, and a variety of salads. Japanese restaurants menu items include vegetable sushi, miso soup, seaweed salad, vegetarian soba noodle dishes and vegetarian rice dishes. Mexican restaurants include bean and rice tortilla with salsa and vegetables, vegetarian chili, salads, bean and vegetable-based soups.

It may not always be possible to research or go to a restaurant that offers plant-based meals, especially when traveling or attending a special occasion that is celebrated with friends or family that still eat meat. But no matter what restaurant is visited, there are usually menu items that can accommodate a plant-based diet. Salads and vegetables that are steamed, baked, or grilled can often be a satisfactory meal for most vegetarians and vegans. It is still necessary, especially for vegans, to ask how the food is prepared so that any animal products used in meal preparation can be avoided.

29. How difficult is it to grocery shop when following a vegan or vegetarian diet?

Thanks to the increasing popularity and demand for plant-based food products, it is just as easy to shop for a plant-based diet as it is for an animal-based diet. Supermarkets offer an increasing selection of vegan and vegetarian food products than ever before. However, many of these foods are processed. For everyone who grocery shops, the ability to read food labels is a must when selecting foods that are healthy. Besides label reading, it is wise to plan a grocery list that includes nutrient dense and minimally processed staple foods, such as dairy alternatives, fruits, herbs, legumes, nuts and seeds, tofu or tempeh, vegetables, and whole grains.

The first step to take before grocery shopping is to write a menu for the week. The menu is the template from which the grocery list is made. Staple foods are included along with special items needed for recipes planned for the week. Because many plant-based foods are processed (see Question 24), it is important to know how to read a food label to select the healthiest and most minimally processed foods available. The Academy of Nutrition and Dietetics publishes a helpful guide about reading food labels in the United States. They recommend the following strategy to better understand how to interpret a food label.

Step 1: Look at the Serving Size

Serving size identifies what is considered to be one serving portion for the food packaged and is the basis for all nutrition information provided on the label. It will also detail how many servings are in the package.

Step 2: Look at Total Calories

This section of the food label reports how many calories one serving size of the food provides.

Step 3: Look at the Percentage of Daily Values

It can be easy to be confused by the individual nutrients and their amounts when looking at a food label. The best way to determine if a food is considered healthy is to look at the daily value (DV) percent reported on the right side of the food label. Daily values are the average amount of a nutrient that a person eating a 2,000-calorie diet should be eating. The percent reported on the food label identifies how much of that food supplies the estimated recommended nutrient need. For instance, a 5 percent DV of fat provides 5 percent of the total fat a person eating a 2,000-calorie diet should eat for the day. When comparing different brands, it is best to find a brand that is 5 percent or less (low) in cholesterol, saturated and trans fats, sodium, and added sugars. These same nutrients are considered too high if they are 20 percent or more and should be avoided. However, good nutrients, such as vitamins, minerals, and fiber, should be greater than 10 percent whenever possible.

Step 4: Look at Nutrition Terms

Food labels have many different definitions and it is important to know what they mean when selecting food items. "Low Calorie" means the serving size is 40 calories or less; "low cholesterol" indicates 20 milligrams or less and 2 grams or less of saturated fat per serving; "reduced" means at least 25 percent less of the indicated nutrients when compared to the nonreduced, original food item; "good source of" provides at least 10–19 percent of the daily value of the indicted nutrient; "excellent source of" means each serving provides at least 20 percent more of the daily value of the indicated nutrient; "calorie free" means less than five calories per serving; "fat or sugar free" indicates each serving is less than half a gram of fat or sugar; "low sodium" means 140 milligrams or less of sodium per serving; and "high in" provides 20 percent or more of the daily value of the specified nutrient per serving.

Step 5: Look for Foods Low in Cholesterol, Saturated Fat, Added Sugars, and Sodium

The goal for good health is to eat less cholesterol, saturated fat, added sugars and sodium. When selecting a food, the goal is select the food brand that is lower in DV of these nutrients.

Step 6: Look for Adequate Amounts of Vitamins, Minerals, and Fiber

Food labels single out the nutrients of calcium, fiber, iron, potassium, and vitamin D because the most current NHANES studies find the average American is deficient in these nutrients. Therefore, food labels include these nutrients to make Americans aware these nutrients are important to include in the daily diet and brands with higher percentages of DV of these should be selected. However, nutrient deficiencies vary from person to person and this section of the label is not always appropriate for some people.

Step 7: Look at Other Nutrients in the Food

It is also important to look at protein if replacing animal protein foods. There is no percentage DV for protein because the amount each person requires for health varies from person to person. Therefore, it is important to know how many grams of protein are needed daily to meet estimated individual requirements. Knowing this figure aids in picking food products that will meet protein needs. Another consideration is the type of carbohydrates in a food brand. Carbohydrates are made of simple and/or complex carbohydrates and sugar. Minimizing sugars and increasing fiber by selecting complex carbohydrates are the best carbohydrate sources to choose. Keep in mind that sugar is found in healthy foods like fruit, which is 100 percent fructose sugar. Fructose sugar is different from glucose sugar, which is found in table sugar or corn syrup, and added to many foods. Fruit should not be avoided because of this, but because it is still a sugar it should be eaten in moderation. One to three servings of fruit are recommended daily. It is important to keep sugars added to a food at a minimum. Looking at the amount of added sugar to a brand is one helpful method when comparing food products.

Besides the food labels, the U.S. Food Allergen Labeling and Consumer Protection Act, also called FALCPA, requires foods that contain major food allergens (i.e., eggs, fish, milk, peanuts, shellfish, soy, tree nuts, and wheat) are labeled in an easy to understand and noticeable way so that consumers are aware of potential food allergens.

A sample whole-food plant-based grocery list is as follows:

Fresh fruits and vegetables
Starchy vegetables: corn, lima beans, peas, potatoes, sweet potatoes, butternut squash
Whole grains: barley, faro, rolled oats, quinoa, whole grain pasta, brown or long grain rice
Healthy fats: avocados, coconut oil, unsweetened coconut, nuts and nut butters, olive oil, seeds

Legumes: black beans, chickpeas, lentils, peas, peanuts, peanut butter
Plant-based milks: almond, cashew, coconut, yellow pea, rice, soy
Plant-based protein: tempeh, tofu, beans, plant-based protein products, soybeans
Spices and seasonings: basil, curry, black pepper, rosemary, turmeric, salt, and so on
Condiments: lemon juice, nutritional yeast, mustard, salsa, soy sauce, vinegar, and so on

If supplementing the diet with some animal foods, include:

Eggs: pasture raised, organic
Poultry: free range, organic
Beef and pork: pastured or grass fed
Seafood: wild caught
Dairy: organic

30. How do I afford a vegetarian or vegan diet on a budget?

While many people think eating a plant-based diet is more expensive than an animal-based diet, most research finds that plant-based diets are actually more economical. Jason L. Lusk and F. Bailey Norwood published a study in the October 2009 issue of *Agricultural and Resource Economics Review* that found in general the majority of plant-based protein was less expensive than animal protein. The only exception to this was the cost of poultry, which was found to be less expensive than corn and wheat but comparable in cost with soybeans. Lusk and Norwood also cited studies finding most plant-based foods are inexpensive nutrient sources and vegetarian diets, in general, reduce food costs.

The following tips can help meet grocery budgeting goals:

Plan ahead.
Dedicating a half hour one night per week to plan menus helps stretch food costs. Keep menus simple and check supermarket flyers for weekly specials that further reduce costs when planning the menu. It is usually best to include three or four favorite recipes that are easy to make and economical, such as black bean burrito bowl, tacos, or baked tofu. Write out a shopping list from the menu and check all staple foods to prevent overbuying foods that may already be in the panty or freezer. This is the most important strategy to stay within a weekly food budget.
Get the best price by comparing and contrasting costs between markets and looking at unit pricing.

Check store flyers, online specials, and local newspapers for sales and coupons. Store loyalty cards can also reduce costs further. Comparing the unit price for brands or different sizes of product is found on the shelf directly under the food item and is the most accurate way to determine which brand or size of the food is the most economical.

Buy fruits and vegetables that are in season or grow them during the spring and summer months.

Stick with whole foods.

Avoid ready-made meals as much as possible. Convenience foods, such as frozen dinners or precut vegetables, are among the most expensive foods in the market.

Shop alone.

Bringing children, partners, or spouses when shopping often results in buying extra food items that cost more and that may not always be the best nutritional choice.

Consider farmer's markets and bulk food stores.

Farmer's markets can be a flexible and cost saving alternative to grocery stores because it is often possible to purchase only what is needed in comparison to grocery stores, where that is not always possible. Another strategy for saving money is to buy foods in bulk. If pantry space allows, purchase bulk items of foods that are used more than once or twice per week and are nonperishable, such as oats, quinoa, rice, canned and dry beans, frozen fruits and vegetables, and spices. Remember, that buying bulk when one rarely eats it does not save money in the long run.

31. What resources are available to support vegetarians and vegans so that meals are flavorful, healthy, and enjoyable?

As vegan and vegetarian diets become more popular, a plethora of nutrition and recipe books, smartphone apps, podcasts, and websites have become available to make transitioning to a plant-based way of life easier than ever before. However, there are many conflicting sources of nutrition information that can be confusing, inaccurate, and sometimes harmful. Whenever any information is sought about nutrition, and specifically plant-based diets, it is important to access established, reliable, and nutritionally accurate sources. While a detailed list of reliable information is provided in the resource section of this book, it is always wise to learn how to evaluate all health care and nutrition information to ensure it can be trusted.

To locate credible, accurate, and helpful information always investigate the source of the information. Any nutrition or health care advice should come from a health care professional that is professionally certified in their respective area of expertise and has worked in their field for a lengthy period of time. One example is T. Colin Campbell who conducted research for the China study and is listed in the resource section. Dr. Campbell completed his education in nutrition, biochemistry, and toxicology and has worked in the field of nutrition research for more than 60 years. He has also taught in many prestigious educational and medical institutions and has collaborated with many other well-established and reputable health care professionals on large-scale human nutrition studies. Always read the "About" section of computer apps, magazines, podcasts, and websites to check the credentials of the author of the information. There are many people who claim to be "nutrition experts" but do not work in the medical or nutrition field or whose advice is only based on their personal experience. Their advice is not always incorrect, but it is not always entirely accurate either and sometimes has the potential to be dangerous for health.

Also, look for well-established and creditable institutions that have served in the medical community for a long time. Institutions such as the Cleveland Clinic, Mayo Clinic, and Harvard School of Public Health are all well-established and respected sources for health and nutrition information based on research and clinician expertise and experience. Foundations and professional organizations are another reliable health care and nutrition resource. Some of these, which also provide plant-based diet topics, include:

The Academy of Nutrition and Dietetics: www.eatright.org
The Academy is the professional organization for food and nutrition
    professionals, such as registered dietitians who are trained to be
    nutrition experts.
The American Heart Association: www.heart.org
Founded by cardiologists, the American Heart Association is dedi-
    cated to fighting heart disease. It is one of the oldest organizations in
    the United States that funds more than $4.5 billion in research to
    decrease heart disease worldwide.
The American Diabetes Association: www.diabetes.org
A professional organization dedicated to reducing the incidence of
    diabetes and funds research to do that as well improve the life of
    diabetics worldwide.
The American Cancer Society: www.cancer.org
An organization of health care professionals who diagnose and treat can-
    cer and also funds research into new treatments and cancer prevention.

Some other organizations that specifically address the needs of vegetarians and vegans are the Physicians Committee for Responsible Medicine, the International Vegan Association, and Oldways Preservation Trust. These organizations provide accurate nutrition information and helpful lifestyle transitioning tips to a plant-based diet and are discussed in the resource section.

32. How can I convince family and friends to accept my plant-based diet choice without alienating them?

Eating meat is a way of life for most people and part of their culture. Animal foods are traditionally included on the menu for many holidays and celebrations, sometimes having religious significance. Sometimes it is difficult for family members and friends to accept an individual's choice to change to a plant-based way of eating.

The majority of people who journey down the plant-based path often do so for health reasons. This reasoning is easier for most people to understand and accept. But individuals who change to a plant-based way of life for animal compassion reasons or because they are concerned about the environment are sometimes thought of as extreme and disrespectful of others who disagree with them. A 2015 study by psychologist Cara C. MacInnis at the University of Calgary, Canada, tested bias toward vegans and vegetarians in comparison to other social groups. She found omnivores perceived vegans and vegetarians more negatively than others with nutritional concerns (gluten intolerance, etc.), especially those who were motivated by animal rights and environmental concerns. The integrated threat theory, which posits a perceived threat leads to a prejudice developing between social groups, may explain the reason for this. In the case of omnivores who eat meat, vegetarians and vegans are perceived as a threat to their attitudes, beliefs, and morals.

Increasing violence against omnivores and animal researchers has not helped the messaging of animal activists either. For instance, Daniel Andreas San Diego, a vegan in California, was placed on the FBI "Most Wanted Terrorist" list for igniting explosive devices outside of biotechnology company Chiron and supplement manufacturer Shaklee in 2003 because they did business with a contract research company that used animals in their research. The FBI cites an increase in violence by animal activists between 1979 and 2008 from organizations such as the Animal Liberation Front (ALF), the Earth Liberation Front, and other extremist groups who committed over 2,000 criminal acts with an estimated

$110 million in damages. Last Chance for Animals president and founder Chris DeRose noted in an interview that the actions of these extremist organizations have actually harmed their peaceful message about animal compassion and has the potential to "set the movement back decades."

Use of animals for research is also increasingly controversial. Scientific researchers are increasingly at odds with animal rights activists, arguing that humane animal research is essential for developing medical treatments for diseases and conditions such as arthritis, cancer, and HIV. A PEW Research Center poll in 2018 found 47 percent of Americans favored using animals in research while 52 percent opposed it. They also found that 63 percent of those with a high level of science knowledge were more likely to support animal research in comparison to 37 percent with medium levels of science knowledge who did not.

The best way to garner the support of friends and relatives when changing to a plant-based diet or way of life is to be mindful about their beliefs. Explaining the reasons for the change in a respectful, understandable manner and without judgment about their eating habits will do more to gain support for an individuals change in lifestyle. Educating others about the documented health benefits of plant-based foods can also promote a healthier lifestyle and diet in others. The 2011 documentary "Forks over Knives" explores the health benefits of changing from animal-based to plant-based diets and may provide one helpful, objective tool to view with family and friends to educate them as to why an individual may be changing to a plant-based diet.

When animal and environmental concerns are the reason for changing, it is extremely important to be respectful and nonjudgmental toward others who still eat meat. Understanding their differing perspective and discussing your beliefs over time, and not preaching about them, will do more to gain support than any other method. Provide objective arguments and resources for them to review if they are interested, but be patient and lead by example. Bringing plant-based recipes to holiday and family/ friend gatherings to showcase how tasty and nutritious plant-based foods can be is another method that may gain their support as well.

33. If a vegetarian or vegan wants to begin eating meat or animal products again, how should they transition to this new diet?

While many people make the transition to eating a plant-based diet successfully and continue to eat this way for the rest of their life, some people do opt to begin eating animal foods again. According to a 2005 CBS News survey conducted by Hal Herzog, PhD, and Morgan Childers, 75 percent of vegetarians transition back to eating meat again. Herzog and Childers informally surveyed 77 ex-vegetarians about their reasons for eating meat again. They found that on average survey respondents had been vegetarians for nine years. Fifty-seven percent became vegetarians because of concerns about the ethical treatment of animals and 15 percent made the choice for health and environmental reasons. Thirty-five percent of respondents cited declining health when on a meatless diet, even though they followed recommended menu plans to ensure adequate nutrition. Twenty-five percent cited the lack of availability of high-quality organic vegetables or the increased prep time needed for recipes. Fifteen percent reported that their plant-based diet decreased their enjoyment of social occasions. Twenty percent reported uncontrollable urges to eat meat again.

The Humane Research Council, also known as Faunalytics, is a non-profit market research organization that studies public opinions regarding animal use. A 2014 study by Faunalytics studied 11,399 American adults. This study found that 83 percent of people eventually abandoned vegetarianism and were older and women. Twenty-nine percent cited health related symptoms and 43 percent cited difficulty following a pure "vegetarian" diet as the reason for transitioning back to an animal-based diet.

For whatever reason, when adding animal foods back into the diet after a period of not eating them, it is best to start gradually to allow the digestive system the ability to adjust and digest animal foods without gastrointestinal distress. The first step to reintroducing animal foods is to eat easy to digest protein foods, such as dairy and eggs. It is recommended that one type of animal food be added to the diet at a time for a few days or taking digestive enzymes to aid the digestive process. Choosing meats higher in fat content can also provide more flavor than other meats, increasing acceptance. For those who struggle with the thought of eating animals again, it may be helpful to consider a social support network to overcome their fear or guilt of eating animal foods.

Case Studies

1. SAM MAKES THE CHANGE TO A PLANT-BASED DIET TO IMPROVE HIS HEALTH

Sam is a 25-year-old male who visited with his primary care physician for an annual health check-up. He is six feet one inch, weighs 300 pounds, and has been feeling well with no health complaints. Sam played football in high school as a linebacker, maintaining his weight around 250 pounds. In the effort to maintain a higher weight than most other players, he developed the habit of eating large food portions, especially of animal protein. Since graduating from college, he works in a job that requires sitting at a desk all day. He tries to be physically active by jogging two miles once or twice per week and working out with weights for an hour three times per week. However, he continues to eat large portions at meals and has gradually gained 50 pounds over the last three years. His daily diet consists of two fast-food breakfast sandwiches and coffee in the morning, two sandwiches and chips for lunch, and grilled meat for dinner with potato or pasta. He doesn't like vegetables but will occasionally eat a salad or broccoli when dining out. Fruit is a favorite snack during the day and he snacks on chips with one two beers at night when watching television. He usually eats pizza, chicken wings, or Mexican food and drinks alcoholic beverages when out with friends during the weekend.

During his check-up, his blood pressure was 140/90. Because a normal blood pressure for his age should be 120/80 or less and he has a family history of heart disease (his uncle died of a heart attack at age 40 and his grandfather died of a stroke at age 55), his primary care physician becomes very alarmed. Sam is also considered to be obese and is approximately 98 pounds over his ideal body weight, putting him an even higher risk for chronic medical conditions and premature death. Subsequently his doctor orders lab tests to further evaluate his cardiac status. The labs ordered include total cholesterol, HDL cholesterol, LDL cholesterol, CRP (C-reactive protein), and triglycerides. Fasting blood sugar and HbA1c labs are also ordered to evaluate for diabetes, since he is over his recommended weight for height and heart disease and diabetes often occur together. Sam's test results come back as follows: total cholesterol 300 mg/dl; HDL cholesterol 40 mg; LDL cholesterol 200 mg/dl; triglycerides 200 mg/dl; fasting blood sugar 150; HbA1c 7.0; CRP: 3 mg/L. All these results indicate that Sam has hypertension, hyper-cholesterolemia, and diabetes that puts him at increased risk for premature death. Sam does not want to take medications and asks his physician if there is anything he can try to reverse these chronic medical conditions. His doctor recommends he work to lose weight and change his diet to a whole food plant-based diet. Since Sam readily admits he is not well informed about nutrition, his physician sends him to work with a registered dietitian and gives him 16 weeks to lose some weight and improve his blood pressure and labs toward the normal range for his age before starting medications.

Sam visits with his dietitian, who reviews his diet habits and eating patterns, analyzes the nutritional adequacy of his daily diet, identifies potential nutrient deficiencies, assesses his weight status, reviews for dietary supplement needs, and formulates an individualized plant-based meal plan for him that is low in fat that will also help him to lose weight. Sam and his dietitian determine that losing weight until he is 200 pounds is a realistic goal for him and a weight he feels he can maintain long-term. He is also advised to increase his exercise to at least half an hour to one hour daily to help him lose weight faster.

Sam faithfully follows the meal plan he is given, although the first two weeks are difficult for him as he adjusts to his new habits. His meal plan and recipes are easy for him to follow and after two weeks he has no difficulties, although he does "cheat a little on weekends" by eating some foods he knows are not healthy and drinking a few alcoholic beverages. Sixteen weeks later, Sam returns to see his doctor who is happy with his progress. At his check-up, his weight is 260 pounds and his blood pressure is 120/80. His labs are as follows: total cholesterol 180 mg/dl; HDL cholesterol 80 mg; LDL cholesterol 75 mg/dl; triglycerides 80 mg/dl; fasting blood sugar 70; HbA1c 5.0; CRP (C-reactive protein): 1 mg/L. Sam's doctor allows him to remain off medications, but he must continue to lose weight and follow his meal plan with regular follow-up appointments to check his progress.

Analysis

It is very common for young men, between the ages of 18 and 35, to eat a diet that is suboptimal in fruit and vegetables and high in protein, calories, fat, sugar, and sometimes alcohol. Former athletes are especially vulnerable because most are encouraged to eat high protein foods and more calories to help them remain competitive within their sport. However, these habits are becoming increasingly common among young women as well. Unfortunately, these dietary habits do not usually change as people grow older and are not as physically active as they once were. Weight gain and diagnosis of chronic health problems at younger ages is increasingly becoming more common and made worse when there is a family history of chronic health conditions. A 2018 study, reported in the AHA journal *Circulation*, found that the rate of heart attacks among young people aged 25–54 is on the rise, especially among women. Diabetes is also being diagnosed more frequently among young people than in the past. Dietary choices, weight gain, and a sedentary lifestyle are the primary risk factors for these chronic illnesses.

To understand the medical urgency for Sam to change his health habits and lifestyle, it helps to know what normal blood pressure and lab values should be for someone in his age range. Blood pressure measures the force of blood flowing through the blood vessels. Two numbers are measured when a blood pressure reading takes place using a blood pressure cuff, known as a sphygmomanometer, and a stethoscope. The systolic measurement (upper number) measures blood pressure at its highest pressure, when the heart contracts. The diastolic measurement (lower number) measures blood pressure at its lowest, when the heart is resting between beats. In 2017, the American Heart Association revised the definition of normal and high blood pressure measurements to lower standards based on the results of the Systolic Blood Pressure Intervention Trial (SPRINT), which found that treatment at lower blood pressure readings than the previous standard of 140/90 reduced the risk for heart attack, heart failure, and stroke. Blood pressure diagnostic criteria for all ages are now defined as:

Normal: 120/80 or less
Elevated: 120–129/<80
Stage 1 high blood pressure (hypertension): 130–139/80–89

Stage 2 high blood pressure (hypertension):
140 or higher/90 or higher
Hypertensive crisis: >180/>120

As we saw with Sam, his blood pressure was 140/90, which places him within the stage 2 hypertension category, significantly increasing his risk for a cardiovascular event.

Besides checking blood pressure, annual physicals include standard lab tests that include a complete blood count to screen for anemia and a complete metabolic panel that screens for heart disease, diabetes, kidney, and liver diseases. Other tests may be ordered when indicated. A lipid blood profile test was included for Sam because of his family background for heart disease. A lipid profile includes checking total cholesterol, low-density lipoprotein (LDL) cholesterol, high-density lipoprotein (HDL) cholesterol, and triglyceride levels. LDL cholesterol measures the amount of "bad" cholesterol in the blood stream. LDL is the main source of plaques that build up in the arteries that may then lead to a heart attack or stroke. HDL cholesterol measures the amount of "good" cholesterol, which helps the body to get rid of LDLs. Total cholesterol measures the combined amount of LDLs and HDLs in the blood. Triglycerides are a type of fat that is found in blood that may increase the risk for heart disease and diabetes. When there is a family history or high risk for heart disease, C-reactive protein (CRP) and very-low-density-lipoprotein cholesterol (VLDL) levels may also be checked. CRP measures the amount of inflammation that may be present within blood vessels. Inflammation is associated with many chronic diseases and illnesses. VLDL measures another type of "bad" cholesterol that has been linked to the plaques that adhere to arteries causing blockages.

The normal values for these diagnostic tests indicating a healthy or normal status are:

Total cholesterol: less than 200 mg/dl
HDL cholesterol: 40 mg/dl or higher
LDL cholesterol: less than 100 mg/dl
Triglycerides: less than 150 mg/dl
CRP: <1 mg/L (>3—high risk cardiovascular disease)

Sam's lab work indicated he was at a very high risk for a cardiovascular event, such as heart attack or stroke. His total cholesterol level was elevated at 300 mg/dl. His HDL cholesterol was 40 mg, within normal range but lower than it should be for someone his age. His LDL cholesterol was elevated at 200 mg/dl. His triglyceride levels were elevated at 200 mg/dl, indicating possible diabetes along with an increased cardiovascular risk. His CRP was elevated at 3 mg/L, indicating a very high risk for cardiovascular disease.

In addition to checking lipid panels during a health check-up, diabetes screening is routinely performed. Diabetes mellitus is one of a group of metabolic diseases that is caused by a defect in insulin secretion, insulin action, or both. Uncontrolled diabetes can cause blindness, vascular disease, limb amputation, kidney failure, and heart disease. Initial diabetes screening tests include fasting blood glucose (FBS) and hemoglobin A1C (HbA1c). To measure FBS accurately, the individual must fast for at least eight hours before blood is taken in the lab, meaning no food or drinks (except water) can be eaten over that period of time. FBS measures blood glucose levels when no food is eaten. If it is normal, but diabetes is still suspected, an oral glucose tolerance test may also be given because blood sugar sometimes rises too high for some people after they eat food, indicating impaired glucose tolerance. The HbA1C is able to measure the average blood sugar level of an individual over the last 6- to 12-week period prior to testing. This is why both FBS and HbA1c are usually both ordered during a routine screen for diabetes. Normal values for FBS are 70–100 mg/dl, and HbA1c are 4–5.6 percent. Sam's FBS was 150 and HbA1c was 7.0, both significantly elevated for his age. These lab results coupled with his elevated triglycerides indicated he had diabetes.

In addition to his lab results, Sam is considered obese, increasing his risk for diabetes and heart disease. Ideal body weight charts became common diagnostic tools in 1959 when the Metropolitan Life Insurance Company formulated standard weight and height tables that defined what a desirable weight for height should be. Ideal body weight is the optimal weight associated with maximum life expectancy for a given height. Healthy weight range became the criteria that was used for individual enrollment in Metropolitan Life's insurance policies and individuals could be denied insurance if they had a significant risk for disease or premature death based on these charts. Updated versions of these charts are still used by medical clinicians today to determine if individuals are at a healthy weight for their height. However, in 1995 the U.S. Department of Agriculture and U.S. Department of Health, Education, and Welfare formulated the body mass index (BMI) measurement, based on NHANES data that identified weight categories that correlated with height and weight charts. This additional criterion is used to define the weight and health status of individuals. BMI criteria are defined as follows:

Underweight BMI: < 18.5
Normal BMI: 18.5–24.99

Overweight BMI: ≥ 25.0
Preobese BMI: 25.0–29.9
Class 1 obese BMI: 30.0–34.9
Class 2 obese BMI: 35.0–39.9
Class 3 obese BMI: ≥ 40.0

According to updated Ideal Weight Charts, Sam's "ideal" body weight should range between 166 and 202 pounds, putting him at 98 pounds over the upper limit of his ideal body weight range. Sam's BMI is 39.6, classifying him as class 2 obesity.

Sam's weight, suboptimal dietary habits, blood pressure, and lab results indicate he is at high risk for an early death unless he loses weight and makes significant changes in his lifestyle and eating habits. Sam's doctor decided to let him try to reverse this health trend through diet changes and weight loss by sending him to work with a registered dietitian. Sam is taught a whole-food plant-based meal plan, which includes low-fat animal foods in moderation, based on the evidence from the China study that indicates he will most likely be able to reverse his current health concerns.

When Sam returns for his follow-up check-up 16 weeks later, his labs have improved significantly and his BMI is 34.3, lowering him to class 1 obesity. This will continue to improve as he loses more weight. His doctor decides to have him continue following his plant-based diet and increased exercise plan without medications. But he must return in six months for a medical check-up to be sure he continues to lose weight and follows his new diet to support the reversal of his potential health problems.

2. MARY BECOMES A VEGAN TO SAVE ANIMALS

Mary is a 15-year-old female who loves animals. One day after school, she attends a seminar that discusses how animals are used for human foods. The video *Food, Inc.*, which explores how food is raised and grown for human consumption, is shown and discussed with the group of attendees. Mary leaves the meeting very concerned about how animals are treated in the food supply chain, especially those that are treated cruelly. She decides to read some books and learn as much as she can about this subject.

After a few weeks, she decides to eliminate all eggs, meat, and dairy from her diet and makes an effort to change to a vegan diet and lifestyle. She feels a little anxious about her decision because some of her favorite foods are hamburgers, fried chicken, cheese, fish, milk, and ice cream. The first two weeks of her new diet are very difficult for her as she eats a diet mostly of vegetables and feels very hungry by the end of her day. But she continues to stick with it and tries to eat more carbohydrate foods to help decrease her hunger. For breakfast she eats a large bowl of oatmeal with added soymilk and fresh fruit. For lunch she eats fresh fruit, a bag of organic potato chips, and a large tossed salad with many different vegetables and added chickpeas for protein. At supper, she often has a veggie burger on a whole grain bun and a glass of soymilk or another salad with chickpeas and lentil soup. She snacks on oatmeal raisin cookies, peanut butter crackers, rice chips, or fresh fruit between meals.

After four weeks Mary is not feeling well. She has lost 10 pounds, feels very tired all the time, and has started to notice some of her hair is falling out. Her mother brings her to see her pediatrician because she is concerned about Mary's eating habits and weight loss. Mary's doctor is immediately concerned that her drastic change in eating habits and weight loss may indicate she has an eating disorder. Unfortunately, many young women with eating disorders use the excuse of eating a meatless diet as a socially acceptable way to hide their disordered eating patterns. He calculates her BMI to be 18.9, which indicates she is still at a normal weight for height despite her 10-pound weight loss (see the case study about Sam for an in-depth discussion of the BMI tool).

However, he discusses his concerns with Mary and sets a specific goal of weight gain that she must reach by her next visit with him in three months. He then orders blood tests to rule out any underlying illness she may have. All of her blood labs come back normal. Her doctor decides to put her on a multivitamin with minerals dietary supplement because her eating habits do not appear to be optimal and she most likely has some vitamin and mineral deficiencies. He also refers her to a registered dietitian for further assessment. During Mary's first visit with her dietitian she is assessed for weight status, whether she shows any indications of an eating disorder, and her current diet habits. Mary's dietitian also requests specific labs that analyze her vitamin and mineral levels and thyroid function, looking for potential nutrition deficiencies. Together they develop a daily meal plan that Mary likes and is able to realistically follow, especially when she is busy with schoolwork or at school events. Her dietitian also supplies her with recipes and websites that she and her family can refer to making meal preparation easier. Mary is encouraged to continue taking her multivitamin with minerals dietary supplement as a way to replete her suspected nutrient deficiencies. Her lab results find she is deficient for calcium, iron, and iodine.

Mary continues to work with her dietitian for two more visits to check that she is gaining weight and her nutritional status is improving as planned. After three months, she returns for a check-up with her doctor, who finds she has regained the 10 pounds she lost, is back to her normal energy level, and is no longer losing her hair.

Analysis

According to Gallup, a market research company, young people aged 18–49 are more likely to follow a plant-based diet for environmental, ethical, and moral concerns.

Faunalytics reports 11 percent of girls, aged 13–17, do not eat animal foods compared to 7 percent of adult women and 5 percent of teenage males. In England, 12 percent of girls, aged 11–16, were reported to be vegetarian. In 2020, Gallup reported American women, aged 18–19, ate less meat than in years past.

However, teenagers and young adults have special nutritional requirements because they are in a period of rapid growth and development. General nutrition guidelines indicate that girls between the ages of 14 and 18 need at least 1,800–2,000 calories and five to six and one-half ounces of protein daily to support growth spurts and developmental needs. Young teen boys, between the ages of 14 and 18, need at least 2,000–3,200 calories and five and one half to seven ounces of protein. Besides calorie and protein needs, mineral and vitamin needs are increased, particularly for B vitamins and vitamin D, calcium, iron, and magnesium. It is quite common for teens to just stop eating animal foods when beginning a plant-based diet, not realizing the importance of replacing nutrients found in these foods from plant sources.

While Mary's weight was normal for her height at her age, weight loss was a concern since eating adequate calories at her age supports growth spurts and muscle and bone development. Regaining the 10 pounds Mary lost was the first goal established as a priority in the short-term. Mary's long-term goal was to then stabilize her weight since she reported she felt good at that weight and she was within her ideal body weight range for her height. Mary was then queried about why she became a vegan and about her current dietary habits. The dietitian was able to rule out a suspected eating disorder as the reason for her major diet changes. Screening for eating disorders is important for all young teenagers, especially girls, who suddenly change their diets as drastically as Mary did. Young girls, but increasingly young men, are under pressure to lose weight and be thin as they become more aware of body image either due to media images, peer pressure, or expectations of a sport that requires a low body weight. The *Journal of the Academy of Nutrition and Dietetics* reported in 2012 that

50 percent of patients with anorexia nervosa followed a vegetarian diet prior to the diagnosis of their eating disorder, compared to 12 percent of those who had no eating disorder history. Sixty-eight percent of eating disorder patients also report that they believed there was a relationship between their eating disorder and vegetarianism, which allowed them to control their obsessively controlled food choices and weight loss in a socially acceptable way.

The next area of concern for Mary's dietitian was to investigate her complaints of hair loss and fatigue. Hair loss is one of the first signs that a diet is not planned appropriately.

When animal foods are eliminated from the diet, there is a sudden drop in protein intake.

As the body adjusts to low protein intake, one of the first things it does is stop growing hair as a way to conserve energy for other vital body functions. When protein loss becomes severe, hair loss will result. Another possible reason for hair loss can indicate an iron deficiency, which also stops hair growth to conserve energy. Since iron is a major nutrient found in meat, especially red meat, hair loss can indicate an iron deficiency. Rapid weight loss also contributes to hair loss because it increases the stress level on the body, disrupting its natural processes. Another concern for Mary is thyroid health. When soy foods are increased in the diet and there is an iodine deficiency (iodine is found mostly in seafood) thyroid functioning may be affected. One symptom of a malfunctioning thyroid is hair and weight loss. Mary's dietitian requested specific labs and found, as suspected, that Mary had some mineral deficiencies. Her thyroid labs were all normal, indicating that her thyroid was still functioning properly, although most likely stressed. Diet analysis also revealed that Mary's protein intake was inadequate and her consumption of processed foods high in sodium, sugar, and fat was excessive. The dietitian educated Mary about vegan diets and how to properly replace critical nutrients found in animal foods from plant sources. Mary faithfully made the changes and successfully improved back to her usual weight and health.

3. ANN VISITS WITH A REGISTERED DIETITIAN TO PLAN A PLANT-BASED DIET TO NOURISH HER UNBORN BABY

Ann is a 30-year-old woman who follows a vegetarian diet. She always ate whatever she wanted until she was a teenager, when she began to vomit every time she ate fish. She was tested and found to have a fish allergy. Other than this, her usual diet consisted of meat and poultry, lots of vegetables and fruits, dairy foods, and whole grain carbohydrates. She did occasionally snack on cookies and chips but always kept her weight stable. She was also active in sports in high school.

One day, when she was 25 years old, she heard on the news that eliminating animal foods from the diet could decrease the risk for heart disease and diabetes. She became interested in learning more about this because she has a family history for both of these chronic illnesses and wanted to avoid developing them as she got older. Before Ann decided to begin a vegetarian diet, she scheduled an annual medical check-up and read the book *Vegetarian Nutrition and Wellness* by Winston J. Craig to learn about nutrition. She learns it is important to replace nutrients that are found in animal foods with those from plant sources to avoid nutrient deficiencies to avoid becoming sick. At her medical check-up, she was found to be at a good weight for her height with no medical concerns. She found the *Vegetarian Starter Kit*, located on the Physicians Committee for Responsible Medicine website, and used this guide to help her transition to a vegetarian diet. This guide provided tips to make her transition easier, recipes, and an eating plan to help her carefully plan her diet to avoid deficiencies.

Ann has maintained good health over the past five years on her vegetarian diet, indicating she planned and implemented her plant-based diet correctly. She continues to be physically active, walking as much as she can when she is at work and working out at the gym one hour a day with weights or on the treadmill. She also maintains a stable weight and feels good. She was recently married and is now expecting a baby. Although she has been healthy, she has read that babies need special nutrients and is worried that her vegetarian diet may increase her baby's risk for birth defects. Although Ann has read some books and looked at websites for nutrition information during pregnancy, she is very confused by all the conflicting advice. She knows that calcium, folate, iodine, iron, omega-3s, and vitamins A, B_6, B_{12}, C, and D are very important nutrients required by a developing baby. She also knows that vitamin B_{12} is found mostly in animal foods and omega-3s are mostly found in seafood. She is unsure if she is eating adequate amounts of these from plant foods and if she should start eating meat again.

Ann would like to remain on a vegetarian diet and discusses her concerns with her doctor. Her doctor is unable to address the nutrition concerns of a vegetarian and only gives her a diet handout that includes animal foods and prescribes a prenatal vitamin. She decides to make an appointment with a registered dietitian who can analyze her current diet and help her to develop a meal plan so that she is eating appropriately during her pregnancy to be sure her baby will be healthy. Prior to her first visit with the dietitian, Ann completes a health history form and food diary for three days. A food diary is a written record of every food and drink and the amounts consumed over a specified period of time. It is used to assess macronutrient and micronutrient intake of the individual being assessed. The dietitian also tests Ann's genomics to learn if she has any gene SNPs (discussed in Question 10) that could possibly impact her absorption for specific nutrients that may impact her health and the baby's. Gene SNPs are genetic variations that can impact a person's health or ability to manufacture necessary enzymes and cofactors the body needs.

Together, Ann and her dietitian review her current nutritional status and increased nutrition needs for a healthy pregnancy. They develop a vegetarian meal plan together that met all of her increased nutrient needs and that she can easily follow. Ann meets with her dietitian one more time to review her nutritional status and diet changes and how she is managing them. Five months later, Ann delivers a very healthy baby.

Analysis

When transitioning from an animal-based diet to a plant-based one, the risk for nutrient deficiencies and insufficient intake of calories and protein is increased when the diet is not properly planned to replace nutrients found in animal foods. As explored in Questions 9, 18, and 19, potential deficiencies for calcium, iron, iodine, omega-3 fatty acids, riboflavin, zinc, and vitamins B_{12} and D are of particular concern for anyone eliminating animal foods from their diet. Young and adult women also have special nutrition needs during their childbearing years to ensure healthy pregnancies with a decreased risk for birth defects. During pregnancy fetal development is rapid, making adequate intake of essential nutrients, protein, and calories critical for proper formation of the fetus. For example, folate is one vitamin that is essential to prevent neural tube defects, such as spina bifida, in the developing fetus. While folate is found in many plant-based foods, it has a symbiotic relationship with vitamin B_{12}, which is primarily found in animal foods. As discussed in Question 20, pregnant women who eliminate animal foods from their diet are at high risk for deficiencies in calcium, folate, iodine, iron, omega-3s, and vitamins A, B_6, B_{12}, C, and D.

During Ann's first visit with her dietitian, the dietitian determines that Ann's weight is within her ideal body weight range and that she is classified with a normal weight BMI. Weight gain recommendations during pregnancy vary for women who are underweight, normal weight, overweight, or obese. The Centers for Disease Control and Prevention (CDC) recommends that a woman within normal weight (BMI 18.5–24.9) like Ann should gain between 25 and 35 pounds during their pregnancy.

   The dietitian then assesses Ann's food diary to determine if she is consuming adequate daily protein to meet both her needs and the growth needs of her baby. Protein needs vary for every individual because protein needs are determined by an individual's weight. Most health care professionals use the U.S. Institute of Medicine Food and Nutrition Board (IOM) recommendations of 0.88–1.1 grams per kilogram of weight to determine the minimum of protein requirements needed per day. The IOM researches and establishes the amount of macronutrient and micronutrient amounts that a healthy person requires to remain healthy. The average protein recommendation for most women of normal weight is 70 grams of protein daily during pregnancy. However, the July 2016 journal *Advances in Nutrition* reported these needs might actually be too low. A small prospective study of 270 women in Vancouver, Canada, where low-birth weight babies rarely occur, used the indicator amino acid oxidation (IAAO) method to determine optimal protein requirements. They found that women might actually need 1.2–1.5 grams of protein per kilogram of weight, or between 78 and 108 grams, per day during pregnancy. Very few studies have been done to date on pregnant women and their nutritional needs, and continued research is still needed in this area. However, Ann's protein intake varied between 75 and 90 grams daily, and the dietitian felt her daily protein intake was optimal during her pregnancy.

   Ann's dietitian then assessed her micronutrient intake, especially for those nutrients that are critical for fetal development. Because Ann still consumes eggs and dairy, the dietitian determines her daily intake of calcium and vitamin B_{12} is adequate. Riboflavin and zinc, which are found in grains, legumes, fortified cereals, and leafy greens, is also determined to be optimal for Ann. However, iodine, iron, and omega-3 intake were assessed to be suboptimal due to the elimination of animal foods and seafood. The dietitian identified good sources for each of these nutrients from plant foods that Ann should be including in her daily diet. Ann's genomic test also showed she had a gene SNP on her FADS1 and FADS2 genes, impacting her absorption of omega-3s. Because of Ann's seafood allergy, an omega-3 dietary supplement made from flax seeds was recommended. The dietitian also recommended a prenatal vitamin mineral combination that ensured all her nutrient needs for a healthy pregnancy were met.

4. BRIAN BEGINS EATING ANIMAL FOODS AGAIN BECAUSE OF ILL HEALTH

Brian is a 28-year-old male who has been following a vegetarian diet for the last six months. Brian's girlfriend started a vegan diet after watching the movie *Food, Inc.*, which discussed how animals are raised for the food supply. She discussed it with Brian, who also watched the movie. They both became more aware of how to eat better for good health. But they also learned about how animals raised for human consumption are treated. They were both particularly concerned about some of the unethical practices used in raising some of these animals. He decided to also follow a plant-based diet, although he did not exclude eggs and dairy.

At the time, Brian was very healthy, and his family had no history of chronic illnesses or food allergies. He is six feet tall and maintained his weight around 150 pounds before he became a vegetarian. His BMI was 20.3 then, classifying him as normal weight for his height. Brian's girlfriend helped him to make the change to his new diet by giving him a copy of the *Vegan Starter Kit* so he can learn how to plan his diet to eat nutritionally balanced meals. She also buys a few cookbooks to cook vegan meals he will like and teaches him to cook these meals for himself as well. Brian finds that he experiences diarrhea and skin rashes any time he eats nuts, oats, legumes, and soy, all foods he never really ate much of before becoming vegetarian. He assumes he is allergic to these foods and avoids them, although he is never tested for this.

Although Brian's girlfriend is doing great health wise on a vegan diet, Brian isn't feeling well since he started his vegetarian diet. Three months after he changed to his new diet, Brian begins to feel very fatigued and just not "quite right" health wise. He begins to gradually lose weight and loses 15 pounds within six months. He continues to struggle to keep his weight stable. His BMI is now 18.3, classifying him as underweight for his height. He also notices that he gets sicker than he did in the past, getting a cold every three or four months. This is even worse during the winter months, when he seems to catch any sickness going around. Brian begins to wonder if he is not eating enough protein because of his allergy to legumes and soy and that he cannot stay healthy on a diet that does not include meat and poultry. He is tired of being too thin, getting frequent colds, having no energy, and not feeling well.

Brian visits with his doctor for a medical check-up. All of his tests and labs come back normal and his doctor tells him to eat more food and think about adding animal foods back into his diet. He begins to add chicken, fish and meat back into his diet, but he feels guilty about eating animal foods again to feel better. In an effort to support the ethical treatment of animals he decides to choose animal food sources that come from farms and other food companies that treat their animals ethically and responsibly.

The first day he adds meat back into his diet, he eats eggs and ham with his breakfast along with whole-wheat toast and fresh fruit, a big hamburger with all the fixings for lunch, and baked chicken with his vegetables, rice, and salad for dinner. He immediately experiences very uncomfortable gastrointestinal symptoms after he eats. However, he continues to eat animal foods every day, although he begins to add them back to only one meal at a time. After a week he no longer has gastrointestinal difficulties. Within a month Brian gains eight pounds and feels increasingly energetic and healthier. After three months he notices he has not had a cold or felt ill. After six months of eating animal foods again, he decides that he made the right decision to add them back into his diet because he is feeling so much better than when he followed a vegetarian diet.

Analysis

While many people remain healthy and thrive on an animal free diet, not all people respond well to the elimination of animal foods, even when they plan their diet optimally to avoid nutrition deficiencies. As discussed in Question 33, 75–83 percent of vegetarians were found to eventually resume eating meat again for a variety of reasons. While it is not yet known why some people do well and some do not on an animal free diet, there are a number of theories including individual genetics, unknown food triggers, health of the gastrointestinal microbiome, or plant substance "toxicity" reactions.

Many adults are unaware they may have a potential food allergy, intolerance, or sensitivity until they are older or increasingly eat a group of foods that they ate infrequently in the past. As reviewed in Question 22, food allergies affect the immune system and symptoms usually appear quickly after eating a suspected food. Food intolerances and sensitivities, however, can affect other body systems besides the immune system with symptoms often appearing days or months later. Any food can trigger a food allergy, intolerance, or sensitivity, but one common food trigger for those eating a plant-based diet is a nickel allergy. Many common plant-based foods are good sources of nickel, a common metal found in the environment, food, and common household items. Brian had experienced diarrhea and a skin rash every time he ate nuts, oats, legumes, and soy. These foods are high in nickel. When he eliminated them from his diet, his symptoms improved indicating he could potentially have a nickel sensitivity.

Besides a possible allergy, intolerance, or sensitivity, genetics may play a role in how well individuals respond to the foods they eat. The genetics a person is born with can affect their ability to digest foods and absorb nutrients properly, via enzyme production controlled by genes, which in turn affects their overall health. One clinician theorizes that our blood type, which carries genetic material, determines the types of food an individual requires to remain healthy. But this theory has yet to be confirmed by studies. Brian's specific genomic make-up was not tested, so it is unknown if his genetics affected his tolerance to a diet low in animal foods. However, since none of his family experienced any negative symptoms from their diets, which included animal foods, it is unlikely his genetics played a role in his intolerance for a meatless diet.

Gastrointestinal (GI) microbiome health, discussed in Question 11, may actually provide more of a clue about why some people do not maintain good health when eliminating animal foods from their diet. As noted, the GI tract is very complex and much more important for good health than ever realized. The bacterial make-up of the GI system affects how well we digest and absorb foods, our immunity, and adequate production of some vitamins, such as vitamins B and K. Brian has never had his GI bacterial health tested so it is difficult to determine if he had bacterial imbalances. However, it appears his immune system is not functioning as well as it should be since he catches colds frequently. This may indicate his GI microbiome health is not optimal. He would be advised to either take a full spectrum probiotic dietary supplement, which contains a wide variety of bacteria known to be beneficial for a well-balanced microbiome, or eat foods that are good sources of probiotics daily. Good sources of naturally occurring probiotics include fermented foods (kimchi, sauerkraut), kefir, kombucha, miso, fermented pickles, sourdough bread, tempeh, yogurt, and some cheeses.

In general, a plant-based diet is high in fiber and it is widely believed that a high fiber diet is beneficial for overall health. However, for some people a high fiber diet can actually cause gastrointestinal intolerance, symptoms of which include bloating, constipation, diarrhea, passing of gas, or intestinal pain. Extreme cases can experience a small bowel obstruction, requiring surgical repair. Eating too much fiber can also increase the transit of foods through the GI tract, decreasing the intestinal tracts ability to absorb calories and important micronutrients, most critically for calcium, iron, magnesium, and zinc. As we saw with Brian, he was experiencing diarrhea, difficulty maintaining his weight, and increased susceptibility for colds. While it initially appears that he could have a nickel sensitivity, he may actually be eating too much daily fiber that could have contributed to his difficulty maintaining weight and diarrhea. Malabsorption of iron and low iron intake from his daily foods could be another reason for his fatigue. Zinc status could also be a problem for him. The mineral zinc plays an important role in good immunity. Low zinc stores, which could result due to rapid transit of foods through his gastrointestinal tract, could also be contributing to his decreased immunity.

One last theory for poor tolerance of a plant-based diet is a negative reaction caused by the defense system found naturally in plants. As Questions 9 and 26 explored, plants have naturally occurring phytochemicals that function as their immune system. Nick did have a negative reaction to oats, nuts, legumes, and soy. It is possible that the compounds found in legumes, nuts, and soy could have affected Nick's intestinal lining, causing his diarrhea. Soy has saponins, which are linked to gut inflammation. Lectins, found in legumes, nuts, and wheat, can also cause intestinal inflammation. These foods could possibly have decreased his absorption of key nutrients, leading to his fatigue. As noted, vegetarians are at higher risk for anemia and Brian did visit with his doctor to evaluate him for anemia or other health conditions.

Once Brian decided to add animal foods back into his diet, he began to eat them immediately with no gradual transition. As a result, he experienced some gastrointestinal symptoms that made him very uncomfortable. Once he slowed his intake of animal foods, he began to tolerate his new diet better with positive health results. But he would have tolerated the transition back to animal foods much easier, and avoided his gastrointestinal distress, if he had done so by slowly adding easy to digest animal foods first and then gradually adding back animal foods one at a time over a few days' time.

5. JOSH'S ATTITUDE ABOUT BEING VEGAN IS ALIENATING HIS FAMILY AND FRIENDS

Josh is a 23-year-old male who read that a plant-based diet is the healthiest and most environmentally beneficial diet to follow. Josh is very healthy and has no health concerns, other than his family has a history of heart disease. He has maintained his weight within his ideal body weight range for his height and at his annual check-ups his cholesterol levels and blood pressure are always normal. However, he has always been concerned about the environment since he was a teenager. Josh is an avid hiker and recently started to volunteer for the Sierra Club, one of the oldest and largest environmental groups in America. He read in *Sierra*, the magazine for the Sierra Club, that raising animals for human consumption increases greenhouse gases that are bad for the environment. He learns, after viewing the United Nations website, that a plant-based diet is one of the best diets to follow to slow environmental warming and help save the planet.

He investigates all the different plant-based diets there are and choses a vegan diet as the best fit for him.

After researching vegan diets, he finds the *Vegan Starter Kit* on the International Vegan Association website. Using this guideline, he is able to learn how to plan his meals nutritionally to remain healthy and transition to his new vegan lifestyle. He also finds cookbooks with easy to prepare recipes that both he and his girlfriend can use to make meals they both like, although his girlfriend does continue to eat meat. Although his girlfriend and family do not agree with his radical change in diet, they try to be supportive of him initially. However, Josh is very passionate about his concern for the environment and is sometimes a little over enthusiastic when talking with his family and friends about it. This has led to many disagreements about how beneficial plant-based diets really are for the environment between Josh, his friends, and his family.

Unfortunately, when Josh goes out with his friends and girlfriend to restaurants, he criticizes anyone who eats a meal with meat. This has caused some serious arguments at the dinner table and many of his friends will no longer go out socially with Josh. His girlfriend will usually avoid meat at meals when they go out, but recently they had a huge argument about going to one of their favorite restaurants because of the restaurants limited plant-based menu options. She is now threatening to break up with him because he is so extreme and is trying to force his choice of lifestyle onto others. His family is also very upset with him. His mother, who is a devout Catholic, has been serving a traditional ham dinner for Easter all of Josh's life. This is a family tradition that is very important to her and their family and has religious significance for them. However, this year Josh is asking that no meat be served at Easter. Josh's mother is very dismayed with his request and is threatening to cancel Easter dinner. His brother and sister have now stopped talking to him because of this request and how saddened his parents are. Josh is very close to his family and is now rethinking his choice to follow a vegan diet.

Luckily, Josh has one good friend who has followed a vegan diet for a number of years. He contacts his friend to discuss his current problems with his family and friends. His friend relates that he went through the same problem when he started. He advises Josh to look for a vegan group in his area on the Internet so he can meet fellow vegans and talk about these issues. Josh finds a local vegan group near his apartment and begins attending meetings. Josh develops a group of new friends that give him advice on strategies he can use when talking with his family and friends to educate them about the environment while also respecting their beliefs and not alienating them. Josh attends Easter dinner, does not criticize anyone, and brings one of his favorite vegan dishes for everyone to try. He also starts to go to restaurants his girlfriend and friends like, planning his meals ahead so that he feels he can remain true to his environmental goals.

Analysis

As we have seen throughout this book, plant-based diets have many positive health benefits. Josh researched the diet before starting it, finding a reliable resource to help him transition to the diet to ensure he ate a well-balanced diet to maintain his good health. Question 31 provides a listing of reliable resources about plant-based diets.

However, navigating his concern about the environment and his change to a vegan lifestyle has been more difficult for him to deal with. As discussed in Question 32, people may feel disrespected and threatened when their way of life is criticized. This in turn often makes them less willing to listen to another individual's perspective about why they have chosen to follow a meatless diet. Unfortunately for Josh, he tended to be very adamant about how bad eating meat is for the environment and criticized the meal choices of others every time he was in a social situation. He was also disrespectful and intolerant of a long-standing tradition within his family, leading to a strained relationship with his family and girlfriend.

As Josh became increasingly alienated from his friends, family, and girlfriend he realized that this was not a situation he wished to continue, even though he remained very concerned about the environment. Luckily, Josh has a friend who is also a vegan and was able to provide good advice that helped Josh continue to live by his ideals while also restoring good relations with his family and friends. Josh began to accept others who ate meat and not criticize them when they ate meat. Instead, he occasionally made comments or suggested resources and movies for his family and friends to watch so they could understand his concerns and why he chose the vegan lifestyle. When he went out to restaurants, he planned his meal choices ahead of time by calling the restaurant or checking their menu online. If the restaurant had limited plant-based entrée choices, he ate a snack before going so that a smaller restaurant meal would be satisfying instead of disappointing. For Easter, he brought a vegan recipe to show his family how good meatless entrées can be and so he also had a meal choice he felt comfortable eating. He also learned to respect and accept the importance of long-standing family traditions of serving meat during special holidays and family gatherings.

Glossary

Animal Rights Movement: social movement that seeks to end moral and legal distinctions between animals and humans and eliminate their use for clothing, entertainment, food, and research

Antinutrients: naturally occurring substances found in plant foods that interfere with absorption or proper functioning of nutrients in the body

Blue zones: five locations in the world where people live the longest and are the healthiest

BMI: body mass index that is used as a screening tool to evaluate the health status of individuals based on their height and weight

China study: research study by T. Colin Campbell that linked chronic illnesses with the consumption of animal foods

Dietary fiber: carbohydrate found in plants that are difficult to digest and aid digestion and removal of food waste from the body

Eating disorders: psychological disorders characterized by abnormal eating habits

Environmentalist: individual who is concerned about and advocates for the protection of the environment

Flexitarian or semivegetarian: individual who eats plant foods and very little animal foods, although occasionally eats chicken, eggs, fish, and red meat

Food allergies, intolerances, sensitivities: abnormal reactions to foods in the diet that can be life altering or life threatening

Genomics: branch of biotechnology concerned with applying genetics and molecular biology to the genetic mapping and DNA sequencing of genes of selected organisms

Greenhouse gases (GHGs): any variety of gases that are believed to contribute to the greenhouse effect by absorbing infrared radiation, trapping it in the atmosphere, and warming the planet

Lacto-ovo vegetarian or lactarian: a vegetarian who also eats dairy foods

Lectins: any class of proteins, mostly of plant origin, which binds to carbohydrates

Macronutrients: nutrients found in foods that provide energy, amino acids, and essential fatty acids that are critical for health, growth, and development

Meat alternatives: a processed food that is similar to meat in protein content but is made from plant sources and used to replace animal protein foods

Mediterranean diet: a diet traditionally eaten in countries that border the Mediterranean Sea that includes primarily plant-based proteins, olive oil, vegetables, and a few animal foods

Microbiome: a community of microorganisms (bacteria, fungi, and viruses) that inhabit a particular environment in or on the human body

Micronutrients: nutrients required in small amounts for normal growth and development of humans

Omnivore: animal or individual who eats both plants and animals for food

Pescatarian: individual who eats only fish for protein and avoids all poultry and red meats

Plant-based diet: diet that includes primarily or exclusively plant food sources, such as fruits, legumes, oils, nuts, seeds, vegetables, and grains; animal foods such as meat, dairy, and eggs are eaten in moderation if at all

Raw food vegan: a vegan diet that only allows raw foods or foods heated to below 104–118 degrees Fahrenheit

Reducetarian: individual who eats less meat and dairy and more plant foods but does not eliminate animal foods from their diet

Vegan: individual who does not eat or use any animal foods or products

Vegetarian: individual who does not eat most animal foods, such as chicken, fish, meat, but does sometimes eat dairy foods and eggs

Whole food: An unprocessed or minimally processed food; both plant-based and animal-based foods can be whole foods

Directory of Resources

Besides resources discussed in Question 31 of this book, the following resources provide reliable guides to help transition to a plant-based lifestyle.

BOOKS

Becoming Vegan by Brenda Davis and Vesanto Melina; 2014, Book Publishing Company, Summertown, TN. https://bookpubco.com/content/becoming-vegan-express-edition

The China Study by T. Colin Campbell and Thomas M. Campbell; 2016, BenBella Books, Inc., Dallas, TX.

A Guide to Vegan Nutrition by George Eisman; 2015, Vegan Publishers, Boston, MA.

How Not to Die by Michael Greger; 2015, Flatiron Books, New York.

The Idiot's Guide to Plant-Based Nutrition by Julieanna Hever; 2011, Alpha Books, Indianapolis, IN.

The Plant-Based Solution by Joel K. Kahn; 2018, Sounds True, Louisville, CO.

Vegetarian Nutrition and Wellness by Winston J. Craig; 2018, CRC Press, Boca Raton, FL.

Whole: Rethinking the Science of Nutrition by T. Colin Campbell; 2014, BenBella Books, Inc., Dallas, TX.

COOKBOOKS

The Beginner's Guide to a Plant-Based Diet by Brandon Hern; 2018, CreateSpace Independent Publishing Platform, North Charleston, SC.

Forks over Knives: The Plant-Based Way to Health by Gene Stone, T. Colin Campbell; 2011, The Experiment, New York.

The Pescatarian Cookbook for Beginners by Daytona Strong; 2020, Rockridge Press, Emeryville, CA.

The Plant-Based Diet for Beginners by Gabriel Miller; 2019, Rockridge Press, Emeryville, CA.

The Vegan Instant Pot Cookbook by Nisha Vora; 2019, Avery Publishing, New York.

MAGAZINES AND PODCASTS

Breaking Down Nutrition by Dr. Susan Mitchell. https://breakingdown nutrition.com

Food and Nutrition Magazine. https://foodandnutrition.org

Sound Bites by Melissa Joy Dobbins. https://www.soundbitesrd.com

SMARTPHONE APPS

Food Monster: Listing of vegan recipes. https://www.onegreenplanet.org /foodmonster/

Forks Over Knives: Provides whole-food, plant-based recipes with cooking instructions and built in shopping lists. https://www.forksoverknives .com/app/

Green Kitchen: A source of healthy vegetarian recipes and cooking instructions. https://apps.apple.com/us/app/green-kitchen/id466252999

The Happy Cow: provides a listing of over 100,000 restaurants that are allergen and gluten free, vegan, and vegetarian friendly. Also posts reviews and menus. https://www.happycow.net/mobile

WEBSITES

The International Vegan Association: https://www.internationalvegan.org

This group of dedicated animal rights activists publishes an online *Vegan Starter Kit* booklet. While the contents of the booklet mostly discuss reasons for becoming vegan, it does offer helpful advice on how to transition to a vegan diet, nutrition guidance, and recipes.

Kaiser Permanente Nutrition Services: https://thrive.kaiserpermanente .org/care-near-you/southern-california/center-for-healthy-living /wp-content/uploads/sites/30/2017/12/Plant-Based-Diet-Eng.pdf

The Plant-Based Diet booklet is provided with reliable nutrition information, menus, shopping lists and tips to start eating plant-based.

Oldways Preservation Trust: https://oldwayspt.org

Very helpful and reliable resource about the Mediterranean diet. Discussion of varying cultural eating habits, vegetarian, and vegan diets. Resources for Mediterranean meal plans and recipes are available.

The Physicians Committee for Responsible Medicine: https://www.pcrm .org

This group of health care providers publishes an online *Vegetarian Starter Kit* booklet that provides reliable nutrition information, recipes, sample diets, and tips on how to transition to a plant-based diet.

T. Colin Campbell Center for Nutrition Studies: https://nutritionstudies .org

Co-author of *The China Study*, Dr. Campbell's website is dedicated to promoting a whole food plant-based diet for good health. The study is discussed along with a "Plant-Based 101" guideline, meal plans, recipes, eating on a budget, and dining out guides.

Vegan.com: https://www.vegan.com

Website dedicated to promoting veganism worldwide, the site provides accurate nutrition information.

Index

About the Author

Alice C. Richer, RD, MBA, LD, is a registered dietitian, certified in advanced functional and genomic nutrition, in private practice in Massachusetts. She is a certified medical writer who has been helping patients improve their nutrition habits and overall wellness for more than 30 years. She received her Bachelor of Science from the University of Rhode Island, Master of Business Administration from Boston College, completed her dietetic internship at the Beth Israel Hospital in Boston, and completed certifications from the American Medical Writers Association, Next Level Functional Nutrition, and Genoma International. She is co-author of *Understanding the Antioxidant Controversy: Scrutinizing the Fountain of Youth* and author of *Food Allergies; A Student Guide to Health: Volume 2, Nutrition and Physical Fitness*; and *Food Allergies and Sensitivities: Your Questions Answered.* You can learn more about Alice on her blog: www.onthecuttingedgenutrition.com